T0355119

Trends and Techniques in Aesthetic Plastic Surgery

Trends and Techniques in Aesthetic Plastic Surgery

Lina Triana, MD
Plastic Surgeon
Clinica Corpus y Rostrum
Cali, Colombia

Elsevier
1600 John F. Kennedy Blvd.
Ste 1800
Philadelphia, PA 19103- 2899

TRENDS AND TECHNIQUES IN AESTHETIC PLASTIC SURGERY,
FIRST EDITION

ISBN: 978-0-323-75710-2

Copyright © 2022 by Elsevier, Inc. All rights reserved.

No part of this publication may be reproduced or transmitted in any form or by any means, electronic or mechanical, including photocopying, recording, or any information storage and retrieval system, without permission in writing from the publisher. Details on how to seek permission, further information about the Publisher's permissions policies and our arrangements with organizations such as the Copyright Clearance Center and the Copyright Licensing Agency, can be found at our website: www.elsevier.com/permissions.

This book and the individual contributions contained in it are protected under copyright by the Publisher (other than as may be noted herein)

Notices

Practitioners and researchers must always rely on their own experience and knowledge in evaluating and using any information, methods, compounds or experiments described herein. Because of rapid advances in the medical sciences, in particular, independent verification of diagnoses and drug dosages should be made. To the fullest extent of the law, no responsibility is assumed by Elsevier, authors, editors or contributors for any injury and/ or damage to persons or property as a matter of products liability, negligence or otherwise, or from any use or operation of any methods, products, instructions, or ideas contained in the material herein.

ISBN: 978-0-323-75710-2

Senior Content Strategist: Belinda Kuhn
Content Development Manager: Ellen Wurm-Cutter
Content Development Specialist: Meghan Andress
Publishing Services Manager: Shereen Jameel
Project Manager: Nadhiya Sekar
Designer: Margaret Reid

Printed in The United States of America

Last digit is the print number: 9 8 7 6 5 4 3 2 1

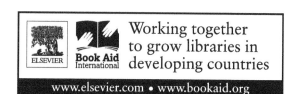

To all our patients; you are the reason why we are here.

Invited Experts

Massimiliano Brambilla, MD
Plastic Surgeon
Milan, Italy

David Caminer, MD
Plastic Surgeon
Sydney, Australia

Gialuca Campiglio, MD
Plastic Surgeon
Milan, Italy

Enzo Citarella, MD
Plastic Surgeon
Rio de Janeiro, Brazil

Fabian Cortinas, MD
Plastic Surgeon
Buenos Aires, Argentina

Waffa Miradmi, MD
Plastic Surgeon
Casablanca, Morocco

Cemal Senyuva, MD
Plastic Surgeon
Istanbul, Turkey

Lina Triana, MD
Plastic Surgeon
Cali, Colombia

Theodoro Vodoukis, MD
Plastic Surgeon
Greece

Preface

In life, many times the easiest way to go is to keep on doing more of the same, but this just does not let us evolve. Evolution comes from opening our minds to new possibilities, new possibilities that open new ways, improved ways on how to do something we thought was just right.

For those who do not know who I am, back in 2007, I became a world pioneer in vaginal rejuvenation procedures. By listening to my patients, I started discovering new possibilities in the world of aesthetic vaginal rejuvenation and how I could really empower women with their sexuality.

Something, that back then was just not considered in our aesthetic practice but today has its own special section in every important meeting all over the world. According to the International Society of Aesthetic Plastic Surgery (ISAPS) world statistics, vaginal rejuvenation procedures are the number one procedure to increase in number when compared to all other aesthetic plastic surgeries in the last couple of years.

So, let us just not stick with what has been written before; let us be open for new—and why not—better ways of doing what we have been doing in our aesthetic field.

We aesthetic plastic surgeons are scientists with high sensitivity for art, and with our artistic minds we are naturally open for these new possibilities, giving us a unique atmosphere for constant evolution and creation in our field.

This book is part of a series where in an easy and friendly interview-with-the-author format, new possibilities will be presented to you. We plan to periodically show you new, better ways to improve techniques and our practices by better serving our patients in the aesthetic world.

All authors with new ideas are welcome to be part of this series!

Lina Triana
Plastic Surgeon
ISAPS President Elect
Cali, Colombia

About the Author

Dr. Lina Triana is a plastic surgeon widely regarded as one of the world's leading experts on the subject of vaginal rejuvenation. Based in Cali, Colombia, Dr. Triana treats patients from all over the world and has been featured in a variety of international media including the BBC. Dr. Lina Triana has been the guest of honor and speaker at more than 50 national and international conferences teaching her colleagues about the latest developments and techniques in vaginal plastic surgery and aesthetic procedures in countries such as Colombia, Venezuela, Peru, Ecuador, Bolivia, Argentina, Chile, Uruguay, Paraguay, Brazil, Mexico, Panama, Guatemala, USA, Canada, France, Monaco, Italy, Belgium, Switzerland, Germany, Greece, Serbia, Rumania, Turkey, Russia, China, Japan, Vietnam, UAE, Lebanon, Israel, India, Tunisia, Egypt, Saudi Arabi, South Africa and Australia.

Dr. Triana is currently president elect 2022–24 of the International Society for Aesthetic Plastic Surgery (ISAPS) and member of its executive committee and board of directors; former president and honor member of the Colombian Society of Plastic and Reconstructive Surgery (SCCP); president 2020–22 of the Colombian Society of Scientific Societies and member of its executive committee and board of directors; international member of the American Society for Aesthetic Plastic Surgery (ASAPS), member of the International Fellowship Committee; member of the International Federation for Plastic Reconstructive and Aesthetic Surgery (FILACP); Honor Member of the Serbian Society for Plastic, Reconstructive and Aesthetic Surgery (SRBPRAS); genital section editor of ISAPS scientific journal, Aesthetic Plastic Surgery Journal (APS); International Editor of ASAPS scientific journal, the Aesthetic Surgery Journal (ASJ); as well as providing multiple scientific input to aesthetic plastic surgery through writing books, book chapters and scientific articles for important aesthetic plastic surgery scientific journals.

Academic degrees: Doctor and Surgeon, Universidad del Valle, Cali, Colombia. Plastic Reconstructive, Maxillofacial and Hand Surgery, Cirugía Plástica, Universidad del Valle, Cali, Colombia. Age Management, Cenegenics Medical Institute, USA. Aesthetic Plastic Surgery, Clínica Interplástica y Clínica Ivo Pintanguy, Rio di Janeiro, Brazil. Aesthetic Medicine, Universidad de Bolivar, Barranquilla, Colombia. Vaginal Rejuvenation and Design, Laser Vaginal Rejuvenation Institute of America, Dr. David Matlock, Los Angeles, USA.

Acknowledgements

To all the authors who made it possible for this book to be published: Thank you to all of you for moving towards something bigger than themselves. When sharing our knowledge, we are acting for the betterment of our specialty, giving the best to our patients, and following our pledge given in the Hippocratic Oath.

Contents

1 Body Contouring with Body Definition Surgery   1

2 Liposuction and J-Plasma   13

3 Mastopexy After Taking Out or Substituting Breast Implants   19

4 A Regenerative Approach to Treat Vulvar and Vaginal Scarring   33

5 Hoodplasty   39

6 Tightening Inside the Vagina   47

7 Scrotal Lift   55

8 Penile Enlargement: Suspensory Ligament, Fat Grafting, Scrotal Webbing   63

9 Fat Grafting to the Penis   75

10 Facial Gender Differences in Nonsurgical Treatments and Treatment of the Tear Trough Deformity   91

Index   101

Chapter 1

Body Contouring with Body Definition Surgery

Introduction Lina Triana Invited Expert

Cemal Senyuva, Plastic Surgeon, Cali, Colombia, Istanbul, Turkey

Chapter Outline

Why Offer Body Contouring Combined With Body Definition Procedures?

Why Is It Important as Doctors to Have Different Treatment Approaches?

Important Anatomical Differences Between Males and Females

Expert Approach: Ultrasonic Liposuction-Assisted High Lateral Tension Abdominoplasty Technique

Why did you decide to do this technique?

When did you learn it or if it is your own, how did you end up doing it?

Can this technique be compared to others and why?

What do you consider are important landmarks and anatomy to be able to better perform this technique?

Can you explain to us how you do the assessment on a patient asking for this procedure?

Can you give us some guidelines for constructing an assessment chart?

Can you describe your technique?

How can we avoid complications?

Can you summarize your follow-up and patient recommendations?

Why do you think this technique should be in the armamentarium of any plastic surgeon?

What tips can you give us to include this procedure in our practice and how to market it?

Expert Profile

In today's world, how we look is important and something that gains more and more attention both for males and females is their body definition. Although physiologically, females have more subcutaneous issue that gives them a more curvilinear look, today's trend of having a more defined look is changing the imaginary ideal for females who today ask also for more body definition. Also, it is important to remember that when there is too much skin laxity, definition is not enough; excess skin also needs to be trimmed.

This is why it is so important for surgeons who do body contouring surgery to have an artistic view and a good knowledge of the normal human anatomy, but it is more important to really listen to the patient so we can end up with realistic results. As surgeons, we must focus on giving the patients the right expectations. Today we do have new technologies that help us achieve better results, but when there is a lot of excess skin with a big abdominal muscle diastasis, more than just liposuction is needed, new technology can help, but it is not magical.

Once again it is important to set the right expectations. If you exam a patient and see that she has a rectus muscle implantation above the rib cage, it will not be right to promise a flat tummy. You can see this in body builders who have no subcutaneous tissue and have extreme muscle definition, and yet many do not have a flat abdomen, so the point is not to think that following the procedure I am going to leave this patient flat, but how I can deliver a natural look, considering the natural anatomy of this individual and our artistic view and taste.

Why Offer Body Contouring Combined With Body Definition Procedures?

Being fit has become an important part of our culture. Fitness is synonymous with health and since many people just do not have a naturally defined body because of their bone and muscle structure, they seek these procedures. Others are simply lazy and pretend to end up with a body-builder's physique with plastic surgery. With today's trend, it is important to not only do body contouring procedures and tummy tucks, but to combine these with body definition options. This is essential in our armamentarium, and so it is crucial to get the knowledge, training, and experience in muscle body anatomy for good natural results.

Why Is It Important as Doctors to Have Different Treatment Approaches?

If we really want to end up with a well-defined body quickly, the easiest way is to sculpt it with liposuction. Other options can be nonsurgical treatments that will not give you immediate definition, but in conjunction with exercise and a balanced diet can help you get to a more fit look. However, when excess skin or muscle diastasis is present, liposuction or nonsurgical devices will not be enough; here, we need to combine procedures such as tummy tucks to end up with better results. We must never forget every patient is unique, and surgery plans need also to be unique to each patient. Performing only a liposuction without addressing excess skin and or loose muscles or performing only a tummy tuck without improving body definition is not what our patients are looking for today.

Important Anatomical Differences Between Males and Females

There are important differences between males and females when addressing body definition. For example, the six-pack in men is more defined and in women, it is more discreet. With women, the shadow is more important; for men, you can go ahead and create a more abrupt indentation. The thorax area is very important in male definition and in women,

the hip–gluteal–back thigh areas are more important. Arms are a great complement for a well-defined body in both men and women.

Let us see what our expert has to tell us.

Expert Approach: Ultrasonic Liposuction-Assisted High Lateral Tension Abdominoplasty Technique

Cemal Senyuva
Plastic Surgeon
Istanbul, Turkey

WHY DID YOU DECIDE TO DO THIS TECHNIQUE?

Although I hold different aesthetic concerns in body shaping in women and men, I basically use the same surgical technique.

I have been using ultrasonic-assisted liposuction and high lateral tension abdominoplasty for over 15 years.

Preoperative drawings of the patients show differences between men and women.

Advanced technical body liposuction teachings and experiences are decisive.

In modern philosophy, body shaping requires three-dimensional shaping rather than two-dimensional.

WHEN DID YOU LEARN IT OR IF IT IS YOUR OWN, HOW DID YOU END UP DOING IT?

In the late 1990s, I learned the technique of high lateral tension abdominoplasty surgery from Ted Lockwood. I started practicing immediately.

In the same years, I received third-generation ultrasonic liposuction training from William Cimino and started to use it.

There was already the necessity of wide and simultaneous liposuction in high lateral tension abdominoplasty, instead of classical technique liposuction. I thought of combining ultrasonic liposuction that emulsifies the fatty tissue selectively and protects perforating blood vessels, connective tissue, nerves and lymphatics better, and I started performing these surgeries in 2003.

In 2010, I hosted Dr. Alfredo Hoyos's HiDef liposuction training in Istanbul and started using HiDef liposuction in body shaping.

With the experiences I have gained from this, I use high-definition approaches and philosophy, ultrasonic liposuction technology, and high side tension technique in the marking and application in body contouring surgeries.

CAN THIS TECHNIQUE BE COMPARED TO OTHERS AND WHY?

Complications are still high in classic abdominoplasty and there are limitations in treating excess fatty tissue. It is difficult to advance the thick flaps and close the wound and to overcome the tension. Aesthetic results may not be satisfactory.

Nonultrasound technologies such as lasers damage the anatomical structures important for tissue circulation in abdominoplasty and are not recommended to be combined. The fat harvested with this technology cannot be used for grafting.

The results obtained with nonsurgical firming or thinning technologies will be suboptimal.

WHAT DO YOU CONSIDER ARE IMPORTANT LANDMARKS AND ANATOMY TO BE ABLE TO BETTER PERFORM THIS TECHNIQUE?

We divide our patients into groups according to their fat pattern and soft tissue laxity. We call the group of patients with skin laxity and low fat accumulation the "skinny patient group." We use ultrasonic liposuction technology for tunneling and minimal aspiration and advance the flaps in an *oblique vector from lateral to medial.*

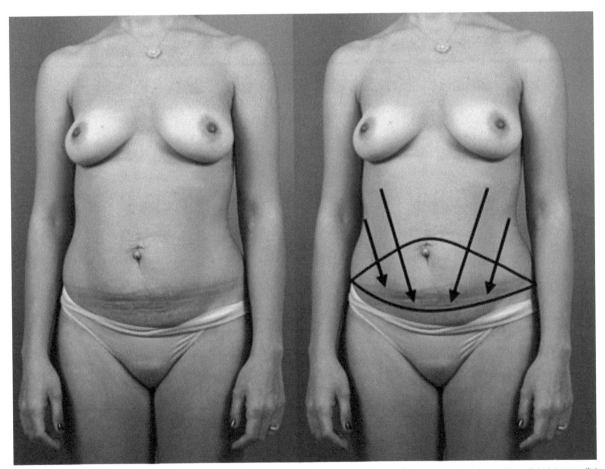

Fig. 1.1 The first group of patients, "skinny patients"; after excision, the upper abdominal flaps will be advanced medially with a slight lateromedial angle.

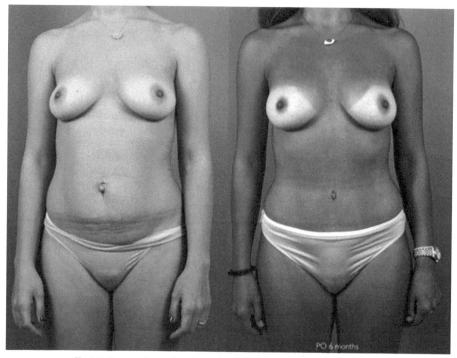

Fig. 1.2 Preoperative and postoperative 6-month anterior view of the patient.

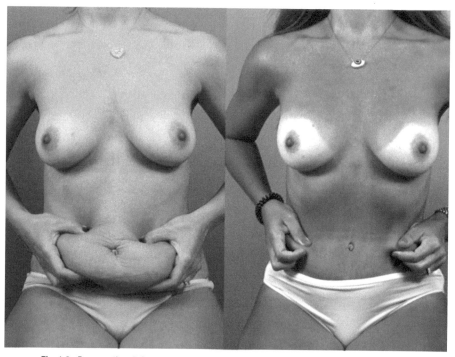

Fig. 1.3 Preoperative *(left)* and postoperative 6-month *(right)* sitting position with rough grip.

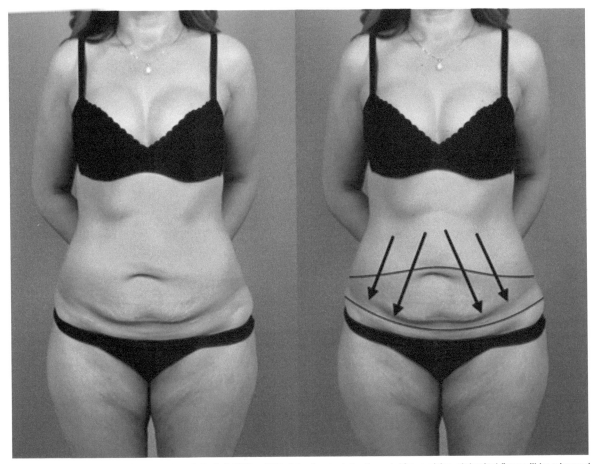

Fig. 1.4 The third group of patients, "epigastric laxity." CAPE or CAP abdominoplasty is planned. After excision, abdominal flaps will be advanced from medial to lateral.

In the second group of patients with fat storage and severe laxity, we use "extended" abdominoplasty marking and techniques. The surgery starts in the prone position with love handle and lumbar liposuction, followed by posterior excision of excessive soft tissue. Abdominoplasty is completed by turning the patient on their back. Advancement and closure with *vertical vectors* are performed in this group of patients.

The third group consists of postbariatric patients. In these patients, cape or pelerin-style planning and technique are applied to correct the epigastric laxity. The flap advancement is performed from *the medial to lateral oblique and outward vectors like a cape*. In this way, the vertical incision and vertical scars of the fleur-de-lis technique are avoided.

Especially in male patients, high-definition surgery can be performed after 6 months following the abdominoplasty.

CAN YOU EXPLAIN TO US HOW YOU DO THE ASSESSMENT ON A PATIENT ASKING FOR THIS PROCEDURE?

The general health status of the patient is questioned. The patient's medical history, previous illnesses and surgeries, smoking habits, allergies, and use of drugs, vitamins, and herbal products are questioned. In female patients, birth control method, pregnancy, and the number of children are questioned. The risk of deep vein thrombosis (DVT) is assessed.

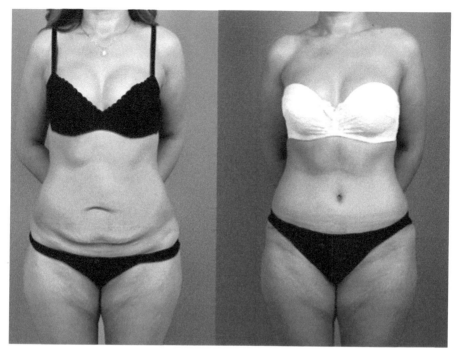

Fig. 1.5 CAP abdominoplasty was performed preoperatively *(left)* and 2 months postoperatively *(right)*.

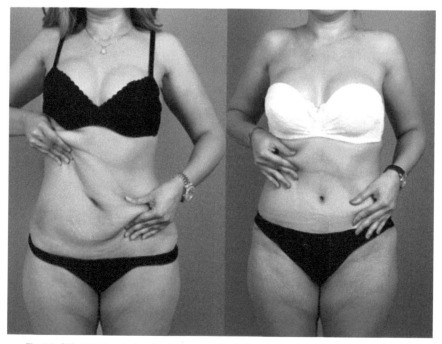

Fig. 1.6 CAP abdominoplasty patient's preoperative *(left)* and postoperative *(right)* rough grip image.

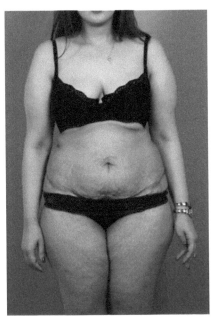

Fig. 1.7 A group of four patients with severe abdominal fat and laxity. Extended abdominoplasty is planned.

Lifestyle is questioned in patients who gain weight and surgery is postponed if there are basic problems related to life habits.

CAN YOU GIVE US SOME GUIDELINES FOR CONSTRUCTING AN ASSESSMENT CHART?

Separate forms can be created for men and women.
The aforementioned issues related to the medical history may be used.
Columns can be created for skinny, extended, and cape group patients.
Body mass index (BMI) and body circumferential measurements can be put in the table.
DVT evaluation can be added to the table again.

CAN YOU DESCRIBE YOUR TECHNIQUE?

A patient is asked to strongly pull up excess tissue in their abdominal region to the maximum degree while the lower incision marking is drawn. This prevents the migration of the incision scar and predicts perfectly its location. In male patients, the incision is planned as

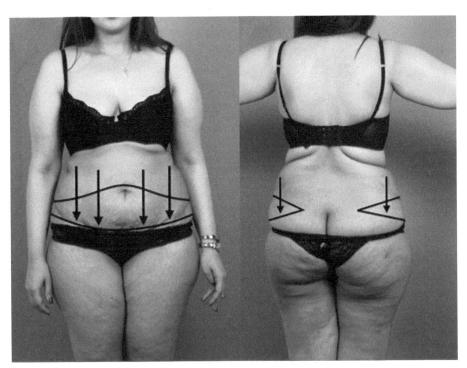

Fig. 1.8 In extended abdominoplasty, flap advancement after excision is performed via vertical vectors. For extended abdominoplasty, the operation is started in the prone position. Back and waist ultrasonic liposuction and posterior wedge excision is performed. The patient is then returned to the supine position for anterior ultrasonic liposuction and excision.

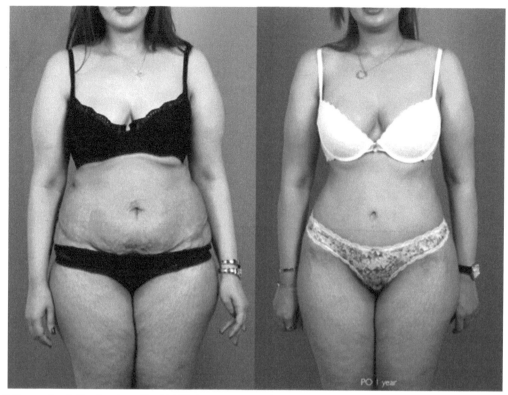

Fig. 1.9 Preoperative *(left)* and postoperative *(right)* first year anteroposterior view of the patient who underwent extended abdominoplasty.

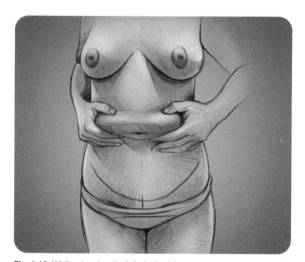

Fig. 1.10 While planning the inferior incision, the patient is asked to pull up all the abdominal soft tissues with both hands. In this way, there will be no scar migration and also, the patient gets a partial lift effect in the groin and upper leg area. The incision site is marked from 6 cm from the anterior vulvar commissure to avoid the abdominal, groin, and leg aesthetic units. A soft curvature facing upwards should be preferred.

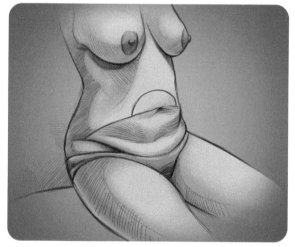

Fig. 1.11 At the end of the marking, the patient is asked to sit down, and the inferior incision line is advanced to the corner of the fold. This will prevent the development of dog-ears.

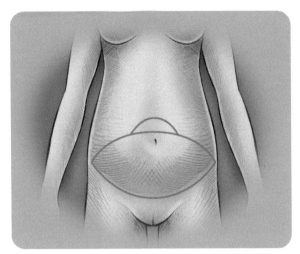

Fig. 1.12 Ultrasound and liposuction should not be applied to the 10 cm diameter semicircular area above the umbilicus. By preserving this area, the flap circulation is protected, and the suprapubic fullness and convexity is maintained after flap advancement.

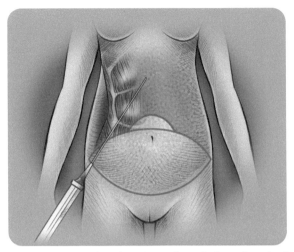

Fig. 1.14 Liposuction is performed according to the three-dimensional shaping concept on axilla, breast lateral, waist, and epigastric areas.

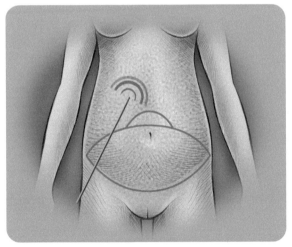

Fig. 1.13 The Klein solution (1,000,000 adrenaline) is infiltrated into all abdominal quadrants except the area to be excised. Skin protection ports are attached, and ultrasonic fragmentation is performed with 3.7 mm probes. The semicircular umbilical area is left intact.

horizontal as possible. In female patients, the marking is shaped like a soft curve facing upwards. The incision should not be within the leg and abdomen aesthetic units.

Secondly, the patient's lipodeposits are marked. The half-moon-shaped area above the umbilicus is protected; this area then provides suprapubic fullness.

Marking for waist depth is done for women, whereas the aim is to protect a square body in men. The mid-epigastric valley, pararectal spaces, subcostal negative spaces, and axillary fat deposits are also marked.

In the first stage of the surgery, Klein solution infiltration is given in the areas where ultrasonic liposuction and excision is planned. After the skin ports are placed, ultrasonic fragmentation is applied with the help of probes.

Liposuction is completed according to the three-dimensional concept. The area is again scrubbed with antiseptic solution.

Open surgery starts by making a lower incision. The incision is deepened to the rectus fascia, trying to reveal the superficial and deep fascias. Dissection is done with electrocautery. In the suprapubic region, the fatty tissue is preserved so that there is no dead space at the closure. The flap is elevated to the level of the umbilicus, making only a narrow tunnel above the umbilicus in the midline, tunnel that is sufficient for making the plication. The umbilical stalk is prepared with scissors. For plication between rectus fascias, 2/0 multifilament nonabsorbable sutures are used. The patient is placed in a semi-sitting position. The umbilical stalk is fixed to the rectus fascia with nonabsorbable sutures. After the flap is advanced, excess tissue is measured and marked with a Lockwood clamp. Superficial and deep fascias are exposed while the excess tissue is excised. The flap is advanced with

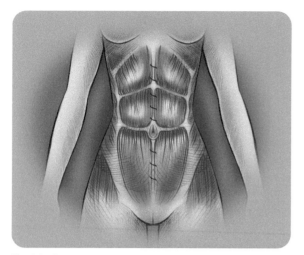

Fig. 1.15 Rectus fascia plication is performed with nonabsorbable monofilament continuous sutures.

progressive tension sutures and the closure tension is minimized. One or two drains are placed according to the liposuction volume. The fascia is closed by continuous suture technique using 3/0 polydioxanone (PDS) barbed suture material on both sides. The skin is covered individually with absorbable separate buried monofilament sutures everting the skin edges. Strips are applied at the end of surgery.

An abdominal binder is applied and closed with moderate pressure. The garment on the lower belly is left loose.

HOW CAN WE AVOID COMPLICATIONS?

Patient selection is important.

Patients with general health problems or who are overweight are not eligible for surgery.

Heavy smokers and candidates who consume excessive alcohol are not accepted.

A psychological evaluation is done. Patients with unrealistic expectations are rejected.

The indication is more selective in women who have not given birth.

DVT precautions should be taken.

Antiembolic socks are used in all patients.

External compression devices are applied and continue to be applied throughout the operation until the patient is mobilized.

Patients are mobilized at the first postoperative hour.

Intravenous (IV) fluid is given to at least 150 ml per hour.

Leg movements are made in the bed.

Megavolume liposuction is prohibited in combined procedures and the amount of liposuction is less than 3 L.

The total duration of surgery is limited to 5 hours.

After a flight longer than 3 hours, patients must wait at least 48 hours before surgery.

Oral contraceptives are prohibited.

Care is taken to protect the perforating vessels to prevent complications of flap circulation during surgery.

The flap is not elevated in areas that are not going to be excised. Laser liposuction is not recommended. Sweeping movements are not allowed with ultrasonic probes and liposuction cannulas.

The corset is not closed under the belly until the circulation is well established, usually after 3–4 days.

Smoking is restricted before and after surgery for a few weeks.

Adequate hydration is achieved with IV liquid.

Tension is reduced with progressive tension sutures while the flap is advanced.

Multiple rotations are not performed for patient positioning during surgery. Only supine and prone positions are used in our practice.

Particular attention is paid to protecting the lumbar region when changing position.

A urinary catheter is not routinely used in male patients.

Preoperative laboratory tests are evaluated together with anesthesia.

If necessary, further laboratory tests and consultations such as endocrine/internal diseases/cardiology/pneumology/hematology are requested.

Surgical site cleaning with chlorhexidine solutions for antisepsis should be done, and it is advised to perform the procedure in highly equipped hospitals. Outpatient clinics and out-of-hospital operations should be avoided. During intubation, 2 g of cephalosporin is given as prophylactic antibiotherapy. No additional dose is given in patients without fat grafting. Rigorous plastic surgical technique and gentle soft tissue handling are essential.

CAN YOU SUMMARIZE YOUR FOLLOW-UP AND PATIENT RECOMMENDATIONS?

Patients stay in the hospital for two nights.

Early mobilization is essential.

Drains are taken out in 48 hours.

The corset is used for 10–14 days depending on the volume of the liposuction and the number of liposuction areas.

Treatments such as lymphatic drainage massages or assisted massage-like machines are not recommended. Patients are check for development of seromas, which are emptied if found.

In case of suspicion for DVT, lower extremity Doppler examination is performed, and parenteral treatment is given when indicated.

Sports are not recommended for at least 3 weeks.

WHY DO YOU THINK THIS TECHNIQUE SHOULD BE IN THE ARMAMENTARIUM OF ANY PLASTIC SURGEON?

Aesthetic results are superior with this technique and approach.

Incision scar location is definite and scar quality is high.

Would healing is very good and complication rates are minimal, thanks to a good patient selection and the postoperative recommendations.

There is a lift effect on the groin area and upper leg.

Abdominal units get thinner in accordance with aesthetic forms.

Male patients may have advanced definition.

Three-dimensional beauty is targeted.

The harvested fatty materials can be used for fat grafts. Breast or pectoral and buttock fat grafting is frequently used in our practice.

WHAT TIPS CAN YOU GIVE US TO INCLUDE THIS PROCEDURE IN OUR PRACTICE AND HOW TO MARKET IT?

It is necessary to invest in an ultrasonic liposuction device and to have proper training with this technique.

Rental facilities are available in some countries.

Apart from participating in training, we recommend learning the technique as an observer.

The literature should be reviewed and kept on file.

Making presentations in congresses, publishing in visual and printed health media, and giving information about the subject on your web page will be enough for promotion.

Expert Profile

Cemal Senyuva
Plastic Surgeon
Istanbul, Turkey

Dr. Cemal Senyuva was born in Istanbul in 1960. He attended Ankara Cumhuriyet High School and graduated as a doctor from Istanbul Medical Faculty in 1983. He began his plastic surgery residency at Cerrahpasa Faculty of Medicine in 1986, where he became a specialist in 1992 and an associate professor in 1997. He taught in the same clinic between 1997 and 2000. In 2007, Dr. Senyuva became professor of plastic surgery in Duzce University Medical Faculty, where he served as head of the Plastic Surgery Department until 2011.

During his early career, Dr. Senyuva worked as Chef de Clinique at Centre Hospitalier Universitaire in Tours, France (1994). He worked as a visiting doctor with Dr. Darina Krastinova at the Foch Hospital in Paris (1994). During 1997 and 1999 he was a visiting surgeon in Paris with Dr. Cornette de St. Cyr, Dr. Patrick Trevidic, Dr. Jean-Claude Dardour, and Dr. Eric Auclair. He was a visiting professor at the Johns Hopkins Hospital in Baltimore, MD, USA, in 1999. In 2001 and 2002, he was a visiting surgeon at Dr. Aysel Sanderson's plastic surgery clinic in Seattle, WA USA.

Dr. Senyuva was the head of the Plastic and Reconstructive Surgery Department at Memorial Hospital, Istanbul, between 2000 and 2003. He was a staff surgeon at Istanbul Surgery Hospital between 2003 and 2007. After serving as the head of Duzce University's Plastic and Reconstructive Surgery Department between 2007 and 2011, he started working full-time in his own private clinic, Istanbul Center. Dr. Senyuva continues to work at his practice today as well as giving lectures, presentations, and leading workshops in Turkey and around the world.

Dr. Senyuva is an expert and a clinical trainer of Ultrasonic (VASER) liposuction surgery, in which he organizes 3–4 workshops a year. To date, he has trained over 30 international plastic surgeons in theoretical and hands-on advanced ultrasonic lipo-suction. Dr. Senyuva is also an International Society of Aesthetic Plastic Surgery (ISAPS) professor, leading instructional courses throughout the year for the ISAPS Educational Council as part of their visiting professorship program. His recent experience includes but is not limited to performing a live operation at ISAPS El Salvador (2016), two live operations at the German Plastic Surgery Conference "Plastische Chirurgie: Kümmern, Kurieren und Kommerz?" in Kassel, Germany (2016), three live surgeries as an invited professor leading an instructional course at the Phuket Plastic Surgery Institute (2016), a live face lift surgery as an ISAPS visiting professor in Ho Chi Minh City, Vietnam (2016), and a live surgery in Linz, Austria (2015).

Dr. Senyuva is an annual speaker at Global Aesthetic Meetings in Miami, FL, USA, and American-Brazilian Meetings (ABAM) in Utah, USA, and Brazil. The most recent conferences Dr. Senyuva was a speaker at include ISAPS Taiwan (2015), the Brazilian-European Synergy's Reshaping the Body Conference in Belgrade, Serbia (2015), XXI Congreso Internacional de la Sociedad Peruana de Cirugia y Reconstructiva in Lima, Peru (2016), ISAPS World Congress in Kyoto, Japan (2016), "A New Horizon in Plastic Surgery" Triangle Plastic Surgical Conference Combined with Annual Meeting of ThPRS and ThSAPS in Hua Hin, Thailand (2016), and the German-Brazilian Aesthetic Meeting "Surf and Curve" in Munich, Germany (2016). He gave three presentations at the XIX International Course of Aesthetic Plastic Surgery and III Symposium ISAPS in Cali, Colombia (2016). He was scheduled to present at the ISAPS course in Amman, Jordan, and at the Global Aesthetic Meeting in Miami, FL, USA (2019).

In 2007, Dr. Senyuva published his book *VASER Abdominoplasty* in English and in Turkish. He has written book chapters in *Omphaloplasty* and *Body Contouring and Liposuction*. He translated chapters from *Grabb and Smith's Plastic Surgery* (6th edition).

Dr. Senyuva is an active member of the American Society for Aesthetic Plastic Surgery (ASPS), Société Française des Chirurgiens Esthetiques Plasticiens (SOFCEP), and ISAPS. He is a past board member and a current member of the Turkish Plastic Reconstructive and Aesthetic Surgery Association (TPRECD), and current president of the Turkish Society of Aesthetic Surgery. Dr. Senyuva currently serves as the chair of the Turkish Plastic Surgery Education Foundation.

BIBLIOGRAPHY

Senyuva C. *VASER Abdominoplasty, Elite Offset.* 2007.
Rubin PJ, Jewell ML, Richter D. *Body Contouring and Liposuction.* 2013.
Murillo W. Omphaloplasty: A Surgical Guide of the Umbilicus. 2018.
Hoyos A, Peres ME, Guarin DE, Montenegro A: A report of 736 high-definition lipoabdominoplasties performed in conjunction with circumferential VASER liposuction, *Plast Reconstr Surg.* 142:662–675, 2018.

Chapter 2

Liposuction and J-Plasma

Lina Triana Invited Expert Waffa Miradmi

Plastic Surgeon, Cali, Colombia, Casablanca, Morocco

Chapter Outline

Why is it Important as Doctors to Offer These Types of Treatments?

Expert Approach: J-Plasma Liposuction

When did you learn it? How did you end up doing it?

Can this technique be compared with others and why?

What do you consider to be important landmarks and anatomy to be able to better perform this technique?

Can you explain to us how do you do the assessment on a patient asking for this procedure?

Can you describe your technique?

How can we avoid complications?

Can you summarize your follow-up and patient recommendations?

Why do you think this technique should be in the armamentarium of any plastic surgeon?

What tips can you give us to include this procedure in our practice and how to market it?

Expert Profile

After liposuction was first described, different techniques and technologies have been invented to assist us during this procedure.

First, the use of tumescent solution was described, which considerably decreased bleeding and the need for transfusions, but still the aim was to decrease fat deposits.

Then an Italian ultrasound device was produced with the intention of liquefying the fat so that it would be easier to extract, but with this technology, complications also started to appear. As this was a power-assisted device, the occurrence of burns in the skin increased. Owing to these complications, the use of this first ultrasound machine was discontinued.

Afterwards, the concept of superficial liposuction was introduced, claiming that better body contours could be achieved, and the term "liposculpture" was first used so that body contouring surgery with liposuction could remove excess fat and put it back where it was missing, so we could truly sculpt the human body.

With this liposculpture technique, skin looseness and irregularities were more commonly seen after the procedure, so there was a need to improve these results and the industry started to work on what options could be available.

We were soon invaded with different power-assisted devices, such as a new ultrasound technology named VASER (vibration amplification by sound energy at resonance) and also different types of lasers, vibro liposuction, and others that would facilitate the surgeon with fat extraction. As many used energy sources that produced heat, this heat could also help with skin tightening.

Today we have a new power-assisted machine that can be used with liposuction called Renuvion powered by J-Plasma. Although not new, use of the

J-Plasma technology for liposuction is a new concept. The manufacturer claims that because the technology was conceived as a cutting device that produced less heat in its surroundings, thereby decreasing burn risks in nearby tissues, this same concept could be extended to liposuction, producing less heat but with much more skin contraction. The manufacturers advertise that the device stating will produce up to 65% more skin contraction.

Why is it Important as Doctors to Offer These Types of Treatments?

Since the invention of liposuction, it has been (together with breast augmentation) the most popular surgical a esthetic procedure done worldwide. As plastic surgeons, we currently all use liposuction and lipoinjection techniques and because we need to be up to date with new scientific advances and innovations, we need to follow and catch up with what technology offers us. However, we can never forget that with liposuction, we are sculpting the human body and by saying so, we are stating that we are sculpting our piece of art in this human body. Although technology will certainly help us improve results or decrease surgery risk, it will never replace the surgeon's artistic taste.

We must not presume that because we buy the newest machine, this will guarantee that we will achieve incredible results, as the end is in the surgeon's hand and the feel of the sculpture being desired as to how successful they will be in delivering the results the patient expects. Therefore, we must stay out of the industry trap that the newest machine will provide better results, as this is not necessarily true. Actually, all these machines that produce heat can increase our surgery risks for complications, especially skin necrosis.

If you have been doing something for, long time and have good and consistent results, why would you want to change it? Many times, we do it because these new technologies can be good for marketing ourselves, making us different from our colleagues, and showing that we are up to date.

In our surgery center, this was the case when we started using laser liposuction, being pioneers in the region in offering this laser-assisted liposuction procedure, Today, we are doing the same by using the J-Plasma

technology in our liposuctions. Different technologies can certainly give us more skin retraction, but we cannot claim it to be consistent with every single case.

J-Plasma technology is a technology that, although new for liposuction, has long been used as a cutting device that claims to produce less heat expansion when used for cutting in surgery. It has very good cutting qualities, similar to those achieved by electrocautery devices, but produces less heat and this is why it was initially thought to be a good option for assisting liposuction. Although it produces heat for skin contraction, because it has a lower heat expansion effect, it would have a lower risk of burning skin.

It is important to know when using J-Plasma technology that helium gas must be infused inside the patient's body so that the J-Plasma can be produced during the procedure. Helium gas does not have any crucial side effects in our body (when used in large quantities it can decrease the percentage of oxygen in the air we breathe), but it is important to prevent its accumulation after the procedure. Therefore, often more incisions for evacuation of the gas are needed, and also it is a good idea to leave incisions open so the gas can leave the body easily after the procedure is finished. Excess gas must also be extracted from the body by "milking" the area towards the incision where the gas was infused, which decreases the excess gas remaining in the body once the procedure is finished.

Currently, I use the Renuvion J-Plasma technology because it can give us a better skin tightening effect, although this is never promised to the patient. Also, we use it because it is a very efficient marketing tool that differentiates us from other plastic surgery practices.

Dr. Wafaa Mradmi is a surgeon who is sharing with us her experience in using this J-Plasma technology.

Expert Approach: J-Plasma Liposuction

Wafaa Mradmi
Plastic Surgeon
Casablanca, Morocco

WHEN DID YOU LEARN IT? HOW DID YOU END UP DOING IT?

I decided to use this technique because I needed a tool that could improve my results, especially regarding the skin tightening after liposuction. I was hesitating between various devices such as laser, VASER, etc., but this one was presented to me as being the best on the market so far, giving the best security and safety in the matter of complications (such as burns).

I started to do the procedure after receiving training by the company that sells the J-Plasma machine – Renuvion – in Morocco, training from a specialist nurse who came from Spain and gave me the basic knowledge on how to operate the machine but was not able to answer many of my questions. As this is a new technology, I knew I would have to learn the details by myself doing my own work while using the device. The one thing that convinced me to buy the technology was that I really "felt" a real retraction of the skin after using the machine during the surgery after having performed liposuction.

CAN THIS TECHNIQUE BE COMPARED WITH OTHERS AND WHY?

As the main purpose of this technique is to improve the skin tightening after procedures such as liposuction or for any loose skin all over the body (face, neck, arms, abdomen, thighs, etc.), yes it can be compared with other technologies that are supposed to give the same results, such as VASER or laser. Although I do not have experience with these other technologies, Dr. Lina Triana, who is familiar with ultrasound liposuction-assisted technology and liposuction laser-assisted technology, says anecdotally that more skin contraction can be seen with this J-Plasma device, although no scientific studies have been done to prove it. All I can say is that you can just see the skin contraction on the operating table.

WHAT DO YOU CONSIDER TO BE IMPORTANT LANDMARKS AND ANATOMY TO BE ABLE TO BETTER PERFORM THIS TECHNIQUE?

The target of this energy is all the fibers that exist between the skin and the muscles that pass through the fat tissue.

It is a blind technique like the liposuction itself and as surgeons, we need to really understand what liposuction is about so in the end, we can proceed to perform the J-Plasma procedure correctly.

As far as I am concerned, I try to do a very safe liposuction (not using the basket cannulas, for example,

that really damage the fibers) when I plan to use the J-Plasma technology.

CAN YOU EXPLAIN TO US HOW DO YOU DO THE ASSESSMENT ON A PATIENT ASKING FOR THIS PROCEDURE?

We are – unfortunately – working in a new era of plastic surgery where patients come into our office asking for new technologies, not just for a technique or even to resolve a physical problem. They just want to solve a problem and because often new technologies are said to give less downtime with good results, this is what people seek more and more today and why they ask for it initially. Here, it is important to tell patients that it is a new device and has only been a few years on the market and not enough data has been collected on its usage.

Because of advertising that we find on Instagram, Facebook, Snapchat, etc., people are aware of a lot of technologies and often presume that they will produce better outcomes. They come to us thinking that the J-Plasma is the solution for their excess skin when the solution is sometimes a good abdominoplasty or facelift.

It is our duty as physicians to explain to them that there are specific indications for this technology, such as moderate loose skin or moderate skin excess, but otherwise, if too much excess skin is present, they will end up with bad results from its technology alone, so when choosing incorrectly by the patient, the device itself will end up having bad advertising.

CAN YOU DESCRIBE YOUR TECHNIQUE?

First, I will do the traditional liposuction and then at the end of the liposuction procedure, I will proceed to use the J-Plasma.

Before starting the J-Plasma procedure, with the cannula under the skin, incisions are interconnected to facilitate gas leaving the body after the procedure. It is important to stop the pass of J-Plasma at least 1 cm from the entrance of the device where the incision is to prevent overpassing it in this area.

The settings I use for the device are as instructed. Sometimes I will raise the power of the device if the skin is thick, and sometimes I will decrease it if the skin is thin (neck, inner thighs, etc.). The average

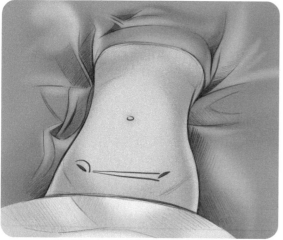

Fig. 2.1 Interconnecting the skin incisions.

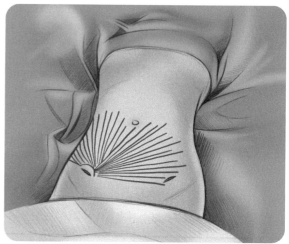

Fig. 2.3 J-Plasma passes done in a fan-like manner.

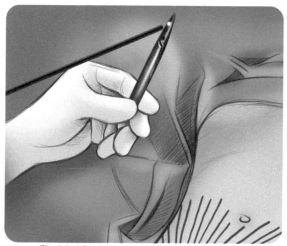

Fig. 2.2 J-Plasma seen when directed to metal tool.

HOW CAN WE AVOID COMPLICATIONS?

If the tightening is really strong after the liposuction, we have to take care about the liposuction itself; It has to be even and uniform; otherwise the J-Plasma will nail the waves more than usual.

We have to be careful regarding how much power is delivered, especially when we treat thin skin areas.

We must not forget that the machine delivers heat and a burn is always possible.

CAN YOU SUMMARIZE YOUR FOLLOW-UP AND PATIENT RECOMMENDATIONS?

I have noticed – and so does the doctor who does the drainage after the liposuction – that we have more edema when we use this technique.

I have increased the number of sessions of post-surgical massages.

I ask the patients to moisturize their skin because they complain about a burning sensation after the liposuction (without any marks on their skin).

I ask them also to keep their girdle around 3 months because of the long-lasting edema, and I tell them to wait for a proper result, which will not be until 8–9 months postoperatively.

WHY DO YOU THINK THIS TECHNIQUE SHOULD BE IN THE ARMAMENTARIUM OF ANY PLASTIC SURGEON?

After months using this device, I have had beautiful results and some average ones (so far).

settings of the machine – Renuvion – are normally for the body, 80 power with 2.0–3.0 of gas release and for the face, 60–70 power with 1.0–2.0 of gas release.

The device is introduced and passes are done in a retrograde linear manner, 1 cm apart from each other in a fanlike manner.

I then do crossed lines, like we do for liposuction, and after I finish the procedure, I put pressure on the skin to evacuate the helium gas that still remains inside at the end of the procedure. Usually two to three passes are done on each treated area. More passes can be done depending on the patient's type of skin and the area being treated.

I am sure that I will reduce and target my indications as I become more experienced in doing this procedure.

Very often, as plastic surgeons, we face challenging cases when a liposuction is not enough and the resection with a big scar is too much. The J-Plasma technology seems to be the solution for those cases, which are not rare in our plastic surgery's practice.

WHAT TIPS CAN YOU GIVE US TO INCLUDE THIS PROCEDURE IN OUR PRACTICE AND HOW TO MARKET IT?

I have to say that it is very rare that I have to inform my patients about this technique, as they have already heard about it. When it is not the case and when I do think that it might be a good option for them, I advise them to consider J-Plasma, explaining to them that it is a new device that will really help with skin tightening.

Expert Profile

Wafaa Mradmi
Plastic Surgeon
Casablanca, Morocco

Although she lives and practices as an a esthetic plastic surgeon in Morocco, Dr. Mradmi is a plastic surgeon who has not forgotten her reconstructive background, participating in over 30 Operation Smile missions and being an active volunteer since 2003 for cleft and palate surgery.

Today, keen to bring the best to her patients, she is one of the first plastic surgeons in her country to introduce the J-Plasma technology into her practice.

WORK EXPERIENCE

From June 2012: Private practice at cabinet MRADMI ALAMI.

From May 2005: Chief of the Service of Plastic Surgery at Hassan II Hospital (Agadir, Morocco) until June 2012.

December 2004: Graduated in Plastic, Reconstructive and Aesthetic surgery (Faculty of Medicine and Pharmacy of Casablanca, Morocco).

1999–2004: Residency in Plastic Surgery at the Service of Plastic Surgery and Burns Hospital, Ibn Rochd, Casablanca. Pr E.H. Boukind (Chief of Service).

1997–1999: Pediatric Surgery (1 year): Pr A. Harouchi (Chief of Service), Internships Dermatology (6 months): Pr H. Lakhdar (Chief of Service), Plastic Surgery and Burns (9 months): Pr E.H. Boukind (Chief of Service).

1990–1996: Faculty of Medicine and Pharmacy, Université Hassan II Plastic Casablanca, Morocco; PhD in Medicine.

PLASTIC SURGERY SOCIETIES

Co-founder of the SOMCEP, Moroccan Society of Aesthetic and Plastic Surgeons
Currently president of SOMCEP
Active member of the SMCPRE, Moroccan Society of Reconstructive and Aesthetic Surgery
Active member of the ISAPS

BIBLIOGRAPHY

Gentile RD: Cool atmospheric plasma (J-Plasma) and new options for facial contouring and skin rejuvenation of the heavy face and neck, *Facial Plast Surg.* 34(1):66–74, 2018.

Gentile RD: Renuvion/J Plasma for subdermal skin tightening facial contouring and skin rejuvenation of the face and neck, *Facial Plast Surg Clin North Am.* 27(3):273–290, 2019.

Kinney BM, et al: Use of a controlled subdermal radiofrequency thermistor for treating the aging neck: consensus recommendations, *J Cosmet Laser Ther.* 19(8):444–450, 2017.

Nelson AA, Beynet D, Lask GP: A novel non-invasive radiofrequency dermal heating device for skin tightening of face and neck, *J Cosmet Laser Ther.* 17(6):307–312, 2015.

Triana L, Barbato C, Triana C, Zambrano M, Liposuction: 25 years experience in 26,259 patients with different devices, *Aesthet Surg J* 29(68):505–512, 2009.

Mastopexy After Taking Out or Substituting Breast Implants

Lina Triana Invited Expert Gialuca Campiglio

Plastic Surgeon, Cali, Colombia, MIlan, Italy

Chapter Outline

Why It Is Important as Doctors to Offer These Types of Treatments?

    Approaches to the area

Mastopexy Technique When Taking Away Breast Implants and Not Replacing Them

Expert Approach: Mastopexy After Taking Out or Substituting Breast Implants

    Why did you decide to do this technique?

    When did you learn it? If it is your own, how did you end up doing it?

    Can this technique be compared to others and why?

    What do you consider to be important landmarks and anatomy to be able to better perform this technique?

    Can you explain to us how do you do the assessment on a patient asking for this procedure? can you give us some guidelines for constructing an assessment chart?

    Can you describe your technique?

    How can we avoid complications?

    Can you summarize your follow-up and patient recommendations?

    Why do you think this technique should be in the armamentarium of any plastic surgeon?

    What tips can you give us to include this procedure in our practice and how to market it?

Expert Profile

When all breast procedures are accounted for, they form a major piece of the pie of all aesthetic plastic procedures performed worldwide. Why? Because breasts are what differentiate males from females.

Throughout art history, we see how important it is for artists to represent the female breast and because plastic surgery is unique among other specialties, regarding the artistic view, this is why for the practice of a plastic surgeon, breast surgery is so important. Although we plastic surgeons are artists of the human body, we surely have important differences from a true artist. An artist is free to make their piece of art; the limit is their imagination. For us plastic surgeons, we definitely have more limitations. We work on human bodies and our starting point is not ideal; this is the magic, we need to make something that is aesthetically consonant, aesthetically balanced. Today, enhancing a person's natural beauty is a must in plastic surgery. The times when plastic surgery was here to show that a procedure was done is in the past, because good plastic surgery today is that which is considered so natural that nobody notices it.

This is why it is becoming more popular to replace large breast implants or even take them out without replacing them, and this is frequently requested in the plastic surgeon's practice today.

As a woman I am more prone to listen to my patients and understand them when they tell me: "Doctor, I wished I had never had the procedure" when referring to their breast augmentation procedure. Cleavage is important not only to reassure our femininity, but also because clothes look better when we have breasts, and here I am not talking about big breasts with deep cleavages.

Once I listen to the patient and understand that she does not wants her implants any more but is afraid of having them removed, I take my time to allow her to understand that doing a mastopexy and not replacing the implants is a good option. However, I tell them I cannot assure a beautiful outcome in the end, as it is not until the implant is out that we as surgeons will see what is truly left of the breast tissue and how much excess skin is present, and can determine how much we can lift the breast and how we can better re-create the upper middle pole, which is what gives the breast cleavage that we like.

By setting the right expectations for the patient, we can proceed in planning to take away the implants without replacing them and to accompany the surgery with a mastopexy.

Why It Is Important as Doctors to Offer These Types of Treatments?

As plastic surgeons, we need to listen and understand what our patients want and design a surgery plan that serves them better.

When taking into consideration taking out or replacing breast implants, many times as surgeons, we believe the patient will end up happier if we leave implants because we will have a better contour, plus the procedure will be easier to perform. However, with years and years of performing these procedures, many times, it can be even easier to take the implants and reconstruct the breast than to reduce the implant or correct malposition of previous breast implants.

APPROACHES TO THE AREA

Whether to remove or replace the breast implants will depend on how and what the patient wants and feels. If the patient tells me, "I am tired of my breast implants," or, "I enjoyed my breast implants, but now they are no longer my priority," *I will propose to perform a mastopexy, remove the implants, and not replace them.*

If the patient says, "For me, it is very important to keep my cleavage. I will not feel good if I lose it," or, "I do not want to lose breast volume; I like my breast size," *I will propose to replace the implants and do a mastopexy.*

Mastopexy Technique When Taking Away Breast Implants and Not Replacing Them

Here I want to share with you my preferred mastopexy technique when taking away breast implants and not replacing them.

1. During the appointment, show Pitanguy's point A to the patient to have an idea of how high the nipple areola complex can move upwards and by doing so, have more realistic patient expectations after the procedure. I always tell the patient, "Please do not forget when you look at yourself in the mirror after the procedure and you think 'I wish they would be higher.'" Remember, as plastic surgeons. We have limitations, and this point A measurement gives us a good idea of how far up the nipple/areola complex can move.

   Point A is estimated by placing your index finger vertically on the submammary fold and projecting it forward and anteriorly on the upper skin of the patient's original nipple areolar complex.

2. The day of the surgery, mark the patient standing up starting with Pitanguy's point A, and also mark the submammary fold.

3. Start the surgery by marking on the operation table a periareolar incision with its upper limit being the previously marked point A. Medial limit of the periareolar incision is no less than 10 cm from the midline and the lateral limit is the lateral aspect of the areola. The lower limit of the periareolar incision is marked under the lower aspect of the areola and can go until 1 cm below, depending on each individual case.

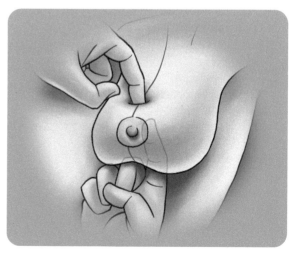

Fig. 3.1 Pitanguy's point A.

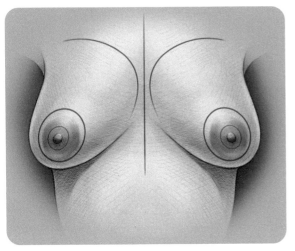

Fig. 3.2 Peri-areolar marking.

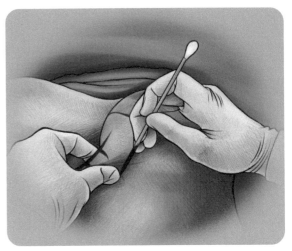

Fig. 3.4 Drawing the vertical limits of the skin resection.

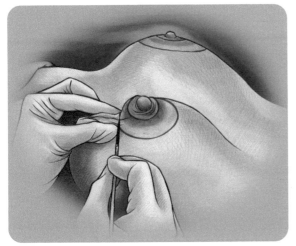

Fig. 3.3 Pinching maneuver to determine the width of skin to be resected.

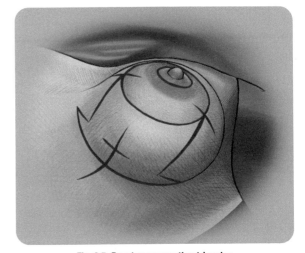

Fig. 3.5 Basal compensating triangles.

4. Afterwards, we make a pinching maneuver on the lower aspect of the periareolar incision and mark where the skin borders touch.
5. Then, two downward vertical lines are drawn, one on each skin mark made with the pinching maneuver. These two vertical lines will be the limits of the skin resection. This skin resection can be widened once the implants are taken out.
6. The vertical lines are measured. They should be between 5 and 7 cm, nearer 5 cm if there is little breast tissue. Basal compensating triangles are marked to match the submammary fold, as seen in Figure 3.5.
7. Marked skin is de-epithelized.
8. We proceed by making a horizontal incision at the submammary fold for extracting the implant. The incision goes through skin, subcutaneous tissue, muscle, and capsule. The implant is taken out through this incision.
9. Dissect the borders of the de-epithelized skin leaving a superior base flap. When needed, resect the implant capsule.

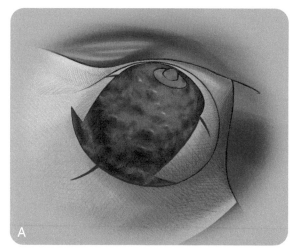

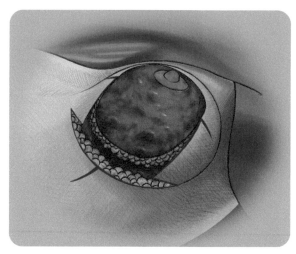

Fig. 3.7 Dissection of the borders of the superior flap.

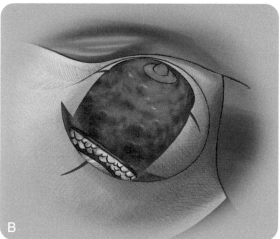

Fig. 3.6 (A) Marked skin is de-epithelized. (B) Incision at the submammary fold for extracting the implant.

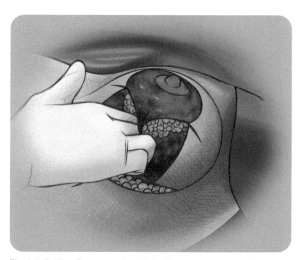

Fig. 3.8 Folding flap upward and fixing it on the medial superior breast quadrant.

10. The flap is folded upwards and 2-0 Prolene sutures are used to fix it on the upper medial breast quadrant to the muscle on the superior limit of the previous breast pocket.
11. Approximation and suturing in layers of the breast tissue and skin is done. If more skin is needed to resect, resection is done before closing the skin. No periareolar purse sutures are done.
12. Preferably, no drains are left; drains increase risk of future skin depression.

Now let us hear our expert and his recommendations on what to do for a mastopexy when a patient wants to have her breast implants taken out or replaced.

Expert Approach: Mastopexy After Taking Out or Substituting Breast Implants

Gianluca Campiglio
Plastic Surgeon
Milan, Italy

WHY DID YOU DECIDE TO DO THIS TECHNIQUE?

I decided to do my technique many years ago when I realized that the traditional approach for mastopexy

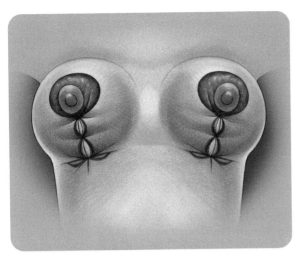

Fig. 3.9 Approximating and suturing tissue and skin borders.

after implant removal or substitution was not appropriate for all cases, and in some circumstances even led to poor results in terms of shape of the breast and reduction of the scar length.

WHEN DID YOU LEARN IT? IF IT IS YOUR OWN, HOW DID YOU END UP DOING IT?

Many years ago, I had the privilege to spend some time with Dr. Claude Lassus from Nice, France, one of the masters in breast surgery. He taught me the basic principles of his mastopexy using the superior pedicle and vertical scar. I was impressed by the simplicity and safety of his technique and I started to use it successfully in my cases of primary breast ptosis and ptosis after implant removal or substitution. In this secondary group, I soon realized that any preoperative marking was difficult or even misleading, as the ideal position of the nipple/areola complex and the distance between areola and inframammary fold (*length of the vertical scar*) were significantly modified after the removal of the breast implant or its substitution. Keeping in mind the principles of Dr. Lassus's technique, I decided to evolve toward a *"free-hand technique"* where the breast mound is created (mastopexy), simulating it with staples or stitches on both sides without removing any piece of skin.

CAN THIS TECHNIQUE BE COMPARED TO OTHERS AND WHY?

My technique belongs to the big family of the superior pedicle breast lifts that have the extraordinary advantage of providing a greater fullness of the upper pole and to prevent a bottoming-out deformity in the long term. It is not an original technique, but rather a mix of these procedures, adopting what I consider the best tips from each of them.

WHAT DO YOU CONSIDER TO BE IMPORTANT LANDMARKS AND ANATOMY TO BE ABLE TO BETTER PERFORM THIS TECHNIQUE?

Some landmarks are important for the correlations of the breast and the thorax, whereas others define the ideal relationships between the different parts of the breast. The former are, for example, the anterior axillary line, the breast meridian, and the midline. The position of the breast on the thoracic cage is also important, as it can occur naturally very low and laterally or medially displaced as in pigeon thorax or in pectus excavatum respectively. The proper breast landmarks are the new position of the nipple/areola complex, the position of the new inframammary fold, and the distance between this fold and the lower border of the areola. Unfortunately, all these references cannot be defined preoperatively with the patient standing because they are conditioned by the presence of the breast implant, and can be decided only after the removal/substitution of the prostheses when the patient is lying on the operating table. Indeed, you could select the ideal position of the nipple preoperatively but once the implant is removed/substituted, this location could be incorrect. This situation makes, in my opinion, the mastopexy after breast removal or substitution one of the most difficult surgical challenges in aesthetic surgery. Ideally, at the end of the operation, the nipple/areola complex should be a little lower than the apex of the breast mound as some inferior dislocation of the breast parenchyma and/or breast implant should be previewed. The distance of the nipple from the sternal notch varies according to the height of the patient and vertical dimension of the rib cage ranging from 17 to 21 cm. One to 1.5 cm above the midline between the humerus and the elbow is another good method to determine where to place the new position of the nipple. What is really important is to not locate the upper border of the areola too high such that it can be seen when a bra or bathing suit is worn. Consider also that too low a nipple areola complex can be easily lifted on a future secondary procedure under local anesthesia after 3–6 months of the primary procedure, whereas an areola that is too high is much more difficult to correct. The position of the inframammary fold is always changed with the mastopexy and can be lowered as in the case of substitution with a large implant or raised as more often happens when the implant is removed or substituted with a smaller one. The ideal distance between the lower border of the areola and the inframammary fold is not fixed as sometimes reported in the literature, but varies according to the final size of the breast, ranging from 5 cm for very small breasts to 8 cm for larger ones.

A sound knowledge of the blood supply of the breast is fundamental, especially in secondary or tertiary cases where a mastopexy has already been performed and vascularization of the areola can be jeopardized by extensive undermining and skin incisions. In primary mastopexy, after implant removal or substitution, the superior pedicle is very safe, even in severe ptosis, providing that the areola is easily inserted in the new keyhole and any tension or compression is avoided. Vascular problems in these cases are always because of a difficulty in the venous drainage rather than reduced arterial perfusion. An accurate preservation of the subdermal plexus can be very useful and helps to prevent superficial slough of the areola in the early postoperative period. In secondary or tertiary mastopexy, undermining is very limited and sometime in case of doubt, a superior and inferior bipedicle can be used for extreme security.

CAN YOU EXPLAIN TO US HOW DO YOU DO THE ASSESSMENT ON A PATIENT ASKING FOR THIS PROCEDURE? CAN YOU GIVE US SOME GUIDELINES FOR CONSTRUCTING AN ASSESSMENT CHART?

In case of *implant removal and mastopexy*, the most important point to be clarified with the patient is if the remaining tissue, sometimes very little, is enough to give her a satisfying volume once the breast is lifted and reshaped. The patient requiring this procedure is often a woman around 50 years old who wants her breast prostheses to be removed because they are old and at risk of rupture, or have already ruptured, and who also desires smaller and more discreet breasts. The use of a fat graft can be taken into consideration when the patient wants a fuller upper pole and a minimal volume increase but refuses a new silicone prosthesis. Of course, the limits of this solution should be

highlighted, mainly the resorption of the fat and the necessity of a sufficient donor site. In selected cases, when more projection and volume is needed, an inferior-based flap of de-epithelialized subcutaneous and breast tissue inserted beneath a superior pedicle (auto augmentation mastopexy) can also be successfully used.

In pure post augmentation cases, a clear description of the location and length of the remaining scars is critical to avoid unhappy patients.

In the case of *implant substitution and mastopexy*, the most critical decision is whether the new prosthesis should be placed in a new implant pocket. Parameters to be considered are the pinch test in superior-medial quadrants (if the thickness of the soft tissue is less than 2 cm a subpectoral placement should be preferred) and the type of result desired by the patient in long-term follow-up. The risk of a waterfall deformity in case of a subpectoral new implant with a significant amount of breast tissue has to be considered and use compared with a prepectoral placement leading to a possible bottoming out, especially if large implants are used. The new shape and volume of the breast should also be discussed with the patient with the help of some postoperative results pictures. A switch from a subglandular to a subpectoral placement of the implant improves the fullness of the upper pole and provides a better coverage of the prosthesis, but at the same time, can make the breasts less mobile and the breast mounds more distant from the midline.

In secondary cases where a mastopexy has already been performed, the increased risk for the vascular supply of the areola should be mentioned to the patient, along with the other typical complications of an augmentation mastopexy.

CAN YOU DESCRIBE YOUR TECHNIQUE?

As previously mentioned, the presence of an implant alters significantly any preoperative marking and drawings, making them inappropriate after the removal of the prosthesis or its substitution, especially if the plane of the pocket is also changed. For this reason, the only references that I mark before the operation are the midline, the breast meridian, and the existing inframammary fold. The procedure starts with a vertical skin incision from the lower border of the areola to a point 2 cm above the submammary fold.

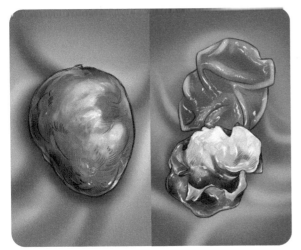

Fig. 3.10 Implant removal with the intact capsule (total capsulectomy). *En-bloc* explantation of an old breast implant with its surrounding capsule. Once opened on the surgical table, the inner calcified layer of the capsule and the ruptures prosthesis are seen.

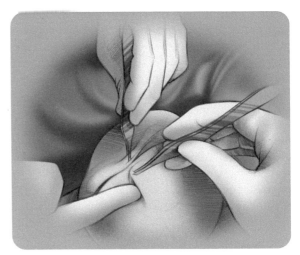

Fig. 3.11 Simulation of mastopexy with provisional stiches.

The soft tissues are dissected up to the periprosthetic capsule and all efforts are made to avoid penetrating it. Breast implants are removed or substituted usually after many years and the risk of dealing with a ruptured prosthesis is very high. The implant therefore is removed together with the intact capsule (total capsulectomy), thus avoiding any dispersion of the silicone gel in to the pocket.

This is very easy when the prosthesis is placed in a subglandular plane, whereas it can be more difficult for the subpectoral implant, especially when the posterior capsule is very adherent to the thoracic wall. Hydro dissection with saline and fine-tip cautery are very useful in these cases. If an accidental laceration of the capsule occurs, the ruptured implant and the gel can be easily removed using a 60-cc syringe without its plunger and directly connected to the aspiration tube. When the implant is substituted, a new pocket is usually created under the pectoralis major muscle unless enough breast tissue is present to adequately cover the prosthesis. Sternal and costal attachments of the muscle must be extensively released to create a nice, regular contour of the infero medial pole. I do not like to transect the muscular belly completely; I prefer to weaken its insertions bluntly, keeping the fascia intact.

At this point, the mastopexy is simulated by suturing the two points that, once closed, correspond to the conjunction of the upper extreme of the vertical scar and lower border of the areola.

The key point of my technique is the simulation of the new areolar opening that is obtained by pinching two points, which once joined will correspond to the conjunction of the upper extreme of the vertical scar and lower border of the areola.

This new areolar opening can be lowered and raised according to the most pleasing appearance of the new

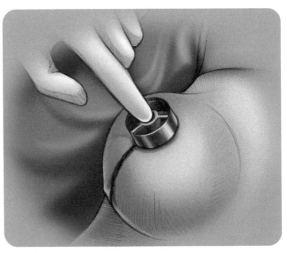

Fig. 3.12 Provisional sutures are removed and skin is excised.

breast mound. Pulling up this stitch, the medial and lateral pillar of the cutaneous resection from the lower pole are shown and are closed temporarily with stitches or staples. With this maneuver, the ideal height of the two pillars and consequently the position of the new inframammary fold are also revealed. The height of the pillars (distance from the areola to the inframammary fold) is not a fixed value but varies according to the final breast volume, becoming gradually greater as the volume of the breast is increased. An internal reabsorbable stitch closes the lower limit of the breast mound approximating the medial and lateral pillars. If more projection is needed, new stitches are used to increase the width of the ventral skin resection laterally and medially until a nice breast shape is obtained. A certain degree of overcorrection is useful, especially in cases of atrophic and relaxed skin, such as in the case of stretch marks. The same procedure is repeated on the contralateral side, following the same steps. Subsequently the symmetry of the two breast mounds is checked measuring the distance of the upper border of the areola from the sternal notch, the medial border of the areola and vertical suture from the midline, and the length of the vertical suture as well. Minor adjustments can be done to obtain the best symmetry in terms of shape and volume and finally, after the

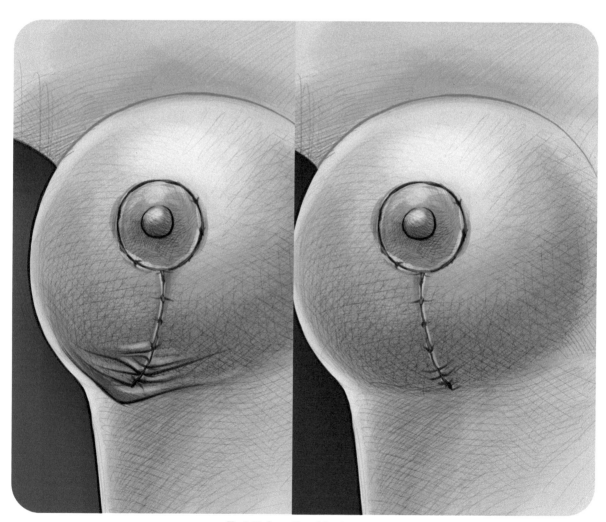

Fig. 3.13 Correction of the dog ears.

marking of the incision lines, the provisional sutures are removed and the skin excised.

Once a satisfying shape of the breast mound is obtained and the symmetries between the two breasts are checked, the temporary stitches are removed and the skin resected.

In mastopexy after implant removal, as much tissue as possible is preserved and in selected cases, a de-epithelized inferior-based flap can be transposed beneath the areola and the superior pedicle. If needed, even the dermis of the flap can be divided, as long as the inferior portion of the transversely oriented septum of the breast is not violated, because the perforators are located along the septum. The inferior dog ear of the vertical suture is defatted with the cautery or liposuctioned and the remaining skin excess gathered with a reabsorbable purse-string suture.

In secondary mastopexy, repositioning of the nipple/areola complex can be done with an oblique vector if its position has been displaced medially or laterally from the midline during the previous operation. In these cases, undermining should be very limited because of the scarring and the increased risk of vascular impairment of the areola.

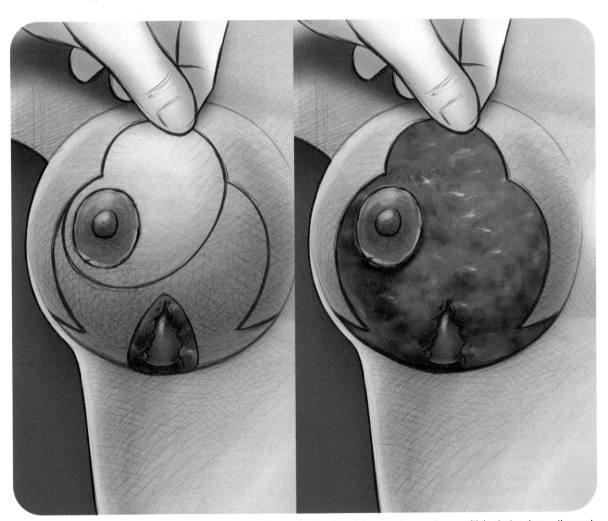

Fig. 3.14 Limited undermining should be done to prevent vascular areolar impairment. In secondary mastopexy with implant exchange, the areola can be laterally or medially displaced so that its repositioning requires an oblique upward movement. In these cases, it is prudent to limit the incisions around the nipple/areola complex to prevent any vascular problems.

HOW CAN WE AVOID COMPLICATIONS?

The most common complications of mastopexy are postoperative hematoma or seroma, wound dehiscence or poor scarring, vascular suffering, or skin necrosis, especially in secondary or tertiary cases. Hematoma incidence can be reduced by the use of drains that require suction in the case of implant substitution. The use of adrenaline solutions is limited to the skin incisions, while deeper infiltrations of the gland are avoided owing to the possibility of a rebound effect. If a hematoma occurs, it should be immediately evacuated as it can interfere with the blood supply of the nipple/areola complex. Seromas can be a result of fat necrosis when an implant is removed in fatty breasts or when a new textured implant is placed in a subpectoral pocket. In the first situation, serum is drained using a syringe or through a small opening in the vertical wound. In the second one, a more aggressive treatment requires bringing the patient back to the operating room and reinserting a suction drain. Wound healing problems can complicate any mastopexy, after either implant removal or substitution and are usually treated conservatively. Of course, in the latter, it is mandatory that the implant is well covered by healthy tissue and that there is no communication with the pocket. Poor scars are revised after 6–9 months, together with other minor asymmetries if present. Superior pedicle is a safe technique in terms of blood supply to the nipple/areola complex, but vascular deficiencies can occur in the very ptotic breast. These are mainly problems of venous drainage as a result of excessive folding of the pedicle. A complete loss of the areola is very rare, whereas partial necrosis or superficial sloughing are more common. They can be treated conservatively with local and systemic antibiotics to prevent any worsening induced by infections. In cases of full thickness loss, debridement can be performed to accelerate the healing process.

CAN YOU SUMMARIZE YOUR FOLLOW-UP AND PATIENT RECOMMENDATIONS?

Following a mastopexy after implant removal or substitution, dressings are removed on the second postoperative day. Patients are allowed to shower and a bra is worn for the following 4 weeks. The inferior elastic band of the bra should be large, at least 1.2–2.0 cm,

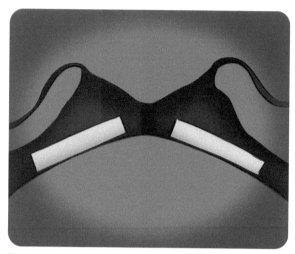

Fig. 3.15 **Adhesive strip of foam to increase pressure on bra.** An adhesive strip of foam is useful to increase the compression of the bra at the level of the new inframammary fold.

and must compress the inferior dog ear of the vertical scar, thus promoting its resorption and the stabilization of the new inframammary fold as well. An adhesive strip of foam can be attached to the bra to increase this pressure.

Arms can be moved immediately after the operation, but exertion and exercises should be avoided for 4–6 weeks. Intradermal reabsorbable sutures do not need to be removed. In some cases of implant substitution, an elastic band over the upper pole of the breast can be useful to prevent an implant displacement. When superficial sloughing of the wound occurs, an antibiotic ointment is used.

WHY DO YOU THINK THIS TECHNIQUE SHOULD BE IN THE ARMAMENTARIUM OF ANY PLASTIC SURGEON?

Mastopexy after implant removal or substitution is a fundamental procedure in the armamentarium of any plastic surgeon because of the great and constantly increasing number of patients who undergo an augmentation mammoplasty. Indeed, according to the most recent International Society of Aesthetic Plastic Surgery statistics, breast augmentation is still the most requested and performed surgical aesthetic procedure in the world. This huge population of patients with breast implants age with resulting modifications of the breast shape and of the implants. Implants have an increased risk of spontaneous rupture that increases with time and this complication scares many women, especially after age 50, so requests to remove the prostheses and reshape the breasts are very common. Also, the breasts age with time, especially if pregnancies or weight loss have occurred, so that a good surgical result can become no longer acceptable and requires a revision even in the case of intact implants. In these patients, mastopexy is effective in reshaping and lifting the breast but often requires also a change of the plane of the pocket and/or the prosthesis to obtain better results.

Secondary or tertiary augmentation mastopexies are not very common, but are very challenging at the same time. These procedures require a simplified surgical approach capable of giving satisfying results in a safe manner. This is achievable with my technique.

WHAT TIPS CAN YOU GIVE US TO INCLUDE THIS PROCEDURE IN OUR PRACTICE AND HOW TO MARKET IT?

My approach is safe and simple, but requires a long learning curve, as preoperative markings are limited and essential. The fact that skin is only removed when the two breast mounds are reconstructed and their symmetry double checked allows the possibility to modify the pattern of the cutaneous resection up until the last moment, thus helping less-experienced surgeons to avoid gross mistakes.

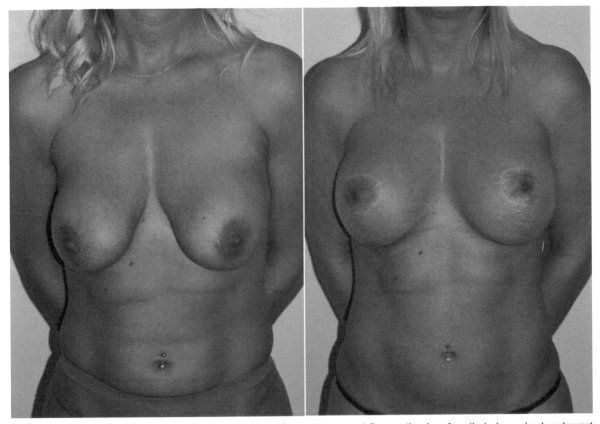

Fig. 3.16 Pre- and postoperative view of a secondary mastopexy after implant removal. Preoperative view of a patient who previously underwent augmentation mastopexy to treat breast ptosis and post-feeding breast deflation. The postoperative picture shows the result after implant removal and secondary mastopexy. In secondary mastopexy the risk of impairment of the blood supply to the areola must be mentioned to the patient along with the other potential complications of augmentation mastopexy.

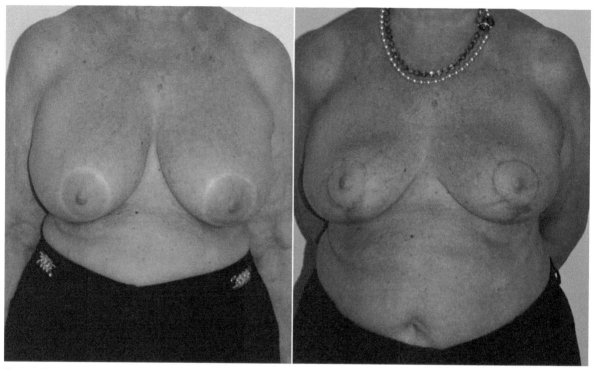

Fig. 3.17 Pre- and postoperative view of a mastopexy after implant and pocket exchange. Patients who underwent subglandular breast augmentation elsewhere through the inferior peri-areolar approach. With time soft tissue coverage reduced and the breasts became ptotic. The postoperative picture shows the result after implant removal, insertion of a larger implant in a new submuscular pocket and mastopexy to lift and reshape the breast tissue.

Expert Profile

Gianluca Campiglio
Plastic Surgeon
Milan, Italy

Gianluca Campiglio concluded his residency in plastic surgery at the University of Milan, where he also obtained his residency in microsurgery and PhD in plastic reconstructive surgery with a thesis on growth factors and stem cells. He has been senior registrar at the Division of Plastic Surgery of Niguarda Hospital (Milan) and consultant in various private and public hospitals. Since 2006 he is only in private practice and is dedicated full time to aesthetic surgery. During his career, he has been author of more than 200 scientific papers in Italian and international journals or books. He is on the advisory board and is section editor of the *Aesthetic Plastic Surgery Journal*. He is 2nd vice president and visiting professor of the International Society for Aesthetic Plastic Surgery (ISAPS), founding member of the Italian Society of Aesthetic Plastic Surgery (AICPE), active member of the Italian Society of Reconstructive and Aesthetic Plastic Surgery (SICPRE), international member of the American Society for Aesthetic Plastic Surgery (ASAPS), and member of the American Society of Plastic Surgeons (ASPS). He has been a consultant for aesthetic surgery for the Italian Health Minister and currently he maintains this position for the Medical Council of Milan.

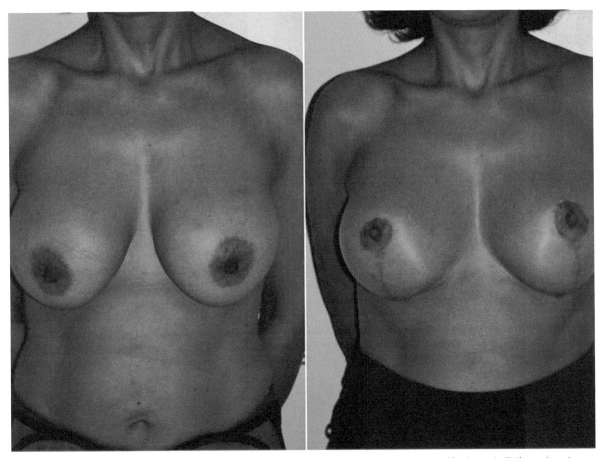

Fig. 3.18 Pre- and postoperative view of a mastopexy after implant and pocket exchange. Another case of implant substitution and mastopexy. The old implants have been substituted by new and larger prostheses inserted in a submuscular pocket. Switching from a subglandular to a subpectoral placement improves the fullness of the upper pole and provides better coverage of the prosthesis but at the same time can make the breasts less mobile and the breast mounds more distant from the midline. A mastopexy reshaped the gland and the skin, repositioning the nipple and areola.

BIBLIOGRAPHY

Candiani P, Campiglio GL: Augmentation mammoplasty: personal evolution of the concepts looking for an ideal technique, *Aesth Plast Surg.* 21:417–423, 1997.

Hidalgo D, Spector J: Mastopexy, *Plast Reconstr Surg.* 132:642e–656e, 2013.

Honig GF, Frey HP, Hasse F, Hasselberg J: Inferior pedicle autoaugmentation mastopexy after breast implant removal, *Aesth Plast Surg.* 34:447–454, 2010.

Lassus C: The Lassus vertical technique, *Aesth Surg J.* 31:897–913, 2011.

Lejour M: Vertical mammaplasty and liposuction of the breast, *Plast Reconstr Surg.* 94:100–114, 1994.

Marchac D: Reduction mammoplasty with a short inframammary scar, *Plast Reconstr Surg.* 77:859–860, 1986.

Nahai F: Current trends in reduction mammaplasty and mastopexy, *Aesth Surg J.* 22:195, 2002.

Chapter 4

A Regenerative Approach to Treat Vulvar and Vaginal Scarring

Massimiliano Brambilla

Plastic Surgeon, Milan, Italy

Chapter Outline

Why Did You Decide to Do These Techniques?

Inevitable scar

True vulvovaginal complications leading to uncontrolled scars

What Is Your Contribution?

Can You Explain to Us the Different Approaches You Offer to Your Patients and the Key Elements for Performing Them?

A regenerative and reconstructive approach to VV scars

VV scar treatment

Episiotomy scar treatment

Vulvar stenosis

Vaginal vault scar after vaginal hysterectomy

TVT mesh erosion/extrusion

Expert Profile

Why Did You Decide to Do These Techniques?

Vulvar and vaginal surgery cause an inevitable scarring process and when major complications occur, an uncontrolled scar process undermines tissue reconstruction. There are inevitable scars and others are true vulvovaginal (VV) complications leading to uncontrolled scars. Here, I explain the differences between these two processes.

INEVITABLE SCAR

Vulvar Surgery

The inevitable subdermal and deep scar as a result of incision and sutures may lead to pain caused by nerve inclusion and tissue distortion. Episiotomy incision, Bartolini cyst removal, and partial vulvectomies are good examples. The loss of issue elasticity determines a dramatic anatomical change, transforming the VV dynamic myofascial system into a rigid and static one. For example, vulvoperineoplasty via fascial plication determines reduction of tissue laxity but determines staticity, increase tissue rigidity, and may determine traction on pudendal nerve fibers located posteriorly to transverse muscle.

Vaginal Surgery

The majority of vaginal surgeries require fixation and controlled scar processes.

Sometimes scars may be painful as a result of pudendal nerve fiber inclusion or traction (e.g., vaginal vault fixation on the sacrospinus ligament after vaginal hysterectomy) or to myofascial abnormal tractions.

Slings and transvaginal tape (TVT) meshes determine a rigid system with often uncomfortable/painful sensations as a result of major loss of tissue elasticity.

TRUE VULVOVAGINAL COMPLICATIONS LEADING TO UNCONTROLLED SCARS

Vulvar Surgery

Hematomas, seromas, infections, and the secondary intention healing process lead to uncontrolled scars.

Vaginal Surgery

Rectovaginal fistulas and urethrovaginal fistulas are among the most challenging complications to fix because of anatomy and poor tissue quality surrounding the fistula.

What Is Your Contribution?

My personal experience is as a result of 22 years of cooperation with gynecologists in a public hospital institution, working together on genital malformations, vulvar cancer, VV stenosis, and atrophies.

The of vulvar and vaginal regenerative surgery are to regenerate tissue, to restore trophicity, to enhance tissue elasticity, and to restore muscle continuity and function.

I have always been looking for innovative regenerative and reconstructive solutions that I share with you today. I will go through different surgical complications of cases such as episiotomy complications, vulvar stenosis, TVT mesh erosions, and vaginal vault scarring after vaginal hysterectomy.

Can You Explain to Us the Different Approaches You Offer to Your Patients and the Key Elements for Performing Them?

A REGENERATIVE AND RECONSTRUCTIVE APPROACH TO VV SCARS

The treatment of the VV scar is based on:
1. Tissue regeneration via fat graft (macro-/micro-/nanofat graft according to tissue damage)
2. Soft tissue reconstruction via flaps for major tissue loss
3. Fascial and muscle continuity reconstruction if possible

To achieve best results, the following points are fundamental:
1. Knowledge of anatomy
2. Knowledge of VV function
3. Knowledge of general fat cell regenerative principles and specific knowledge of genital fat graft
4. Knowledge of genital tissue expansion/distraction and pelvic floor rehabilitation

VV SCAR TREATMENT

1. EPISIOTOMY SCAR
2. VULVAR STENOSIS
3. TVT MESH EROSION/EXTRUSION
4. VAGINAL VAULT SCAR AFTER VAGINAL HYSTERECTOMY

EPISIOTOMY SCAR TREATMENT

INDICATION: vulvar pain after episiotomy scar nonresponsive to pelvic floor rehabilitation
  SURGICAL STRATEGY:
  • HOSPITALIZATION: day surgery
  • ANESTHESIA: nerve blocks + local + sedation
  • ARMAMENTARIUM: microfat graft kit, 18-gauge needle for rigotomies (percutaneous scar release), surgical instruments (if needed)
  • SURGICAL PLAN:
    a. no major loss of tissue (<3 cm of tissue loss between ideal medial vulvar wall line and defect)
      · Microfat graft + rigotomies: Starting from the subdermal area, microfat grafts are placed medially via percutaneous release, reaching most lateral scar tissues. Fat quality: decanted microfat graft (to have fluid graft that can expand tissues) Quantities: 5–15 cc according to tissue damage extension
    b. major tissue loss (>3 cm of tissue loss between ideal medial vulvar wall line and defect)
      · incision of the episiotomy scar, open wound microfat graft + rigotomies + perineal island flap inset

In most cases, one single session is enough to achieve good functional results. An additional fat graft procedure may be necessary at 4 months after the primary surgery.

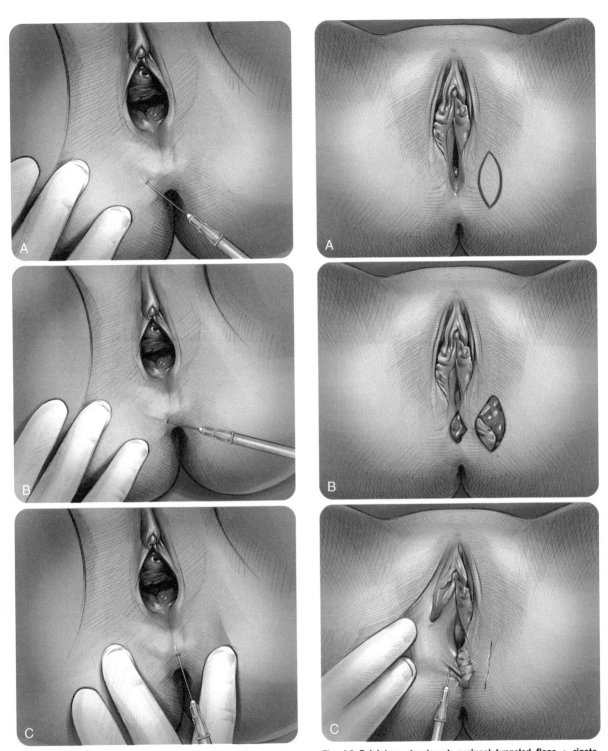

Fig. 4.1 Episiotomy treatment: rigotomies + microfat graft. (A) Superficial scar release. (B) Deep fat release. (C) Perineal fat release.

Fig. 4.2 Episiotomy treatment: perineal tunneled flaps + rigotomies + microfat graft. (A) Flap markings. (B) Dissection and flap tunneling. (C) Closure + riogotomies + microfat graft.

- POSTOPERATIVE INDICATIONS
  - 10 days postoperatively, the patient is encouraged to start massage of the vulvar introitus with cream.
  - 15 days postoperatively, the patient will start expanding the vulvar area via an expandable intruder twice a day for 10 minutes for 2 months.

VULVAR STENOSIS

INDICATIONS:
a. high-degree stenosis (total or subtotal stenosis, impossible inspection)
b. medium-degree stenosis (impossible sexual intercourse, difficult inspection)
c. low-degree stenosis with recurrent ulceration at posterior commissure

SURGICAL STRATEGY:
- HOSPITALIZATION: day surgery
- ANESTHESIA: nerve blocks+ local + sedation
- ARMAMENTARIUM: microfat graft kit, 18-gauge needle for rigotomies (percutaneous scar release), surgical instruments (if needed)
- SURGICAL PLAN:
  a. TYPE A: Incision is carried out along vulvar pillars and posterior commissure to open the introitus as much as possible. Open wound microfat graft + rigotomies are performed in the wound and in the perineal and superior vulvar portion. An extended labia majora double-island flap is tunneled under the vulvar skin bridge.
  b. TYPE B: Incision is carried out along inferior portion of the vulvar pillars and posterior commissure. Open wound microfat graft + rigotomies are performed in the wound and in the perineal and superior vulvar portion. A double-perineal island flap is tunneled under the vulvar skin bridge and sutured medially.

  TYPE C: Microfat graft + rigotomies are performed extensively on the vulvar pillar to commissure and in the perineal area. Fat quality: decanted microfat graft (to have fluid graft that can expand tissues). Quantities: 10–15 cc according to extension of the stenosis.
- POSTOPERATIVE INDICATIONS
  - 10 days postoperatively, the patient is encouraged to start massage of the vulvar introitus with cream.
  - 15 days postoperatively, the patient will start expanding the vulvar area via an expandable intruder twice a day for 10 minutes for 2 months.

KEY TRICKS
1. Rigotomies + microfat grafting can be done intraoperatively via the open wound.
2. Home postoperative expansion is key.

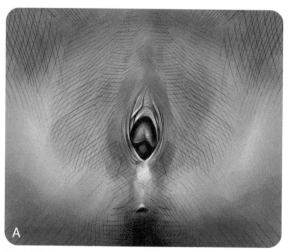 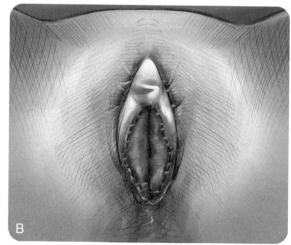

Fig. 4.3 Rigotomy microfat graft + labia majora island tunneled flaps. (A) Preoperative. (B) Postoperative.

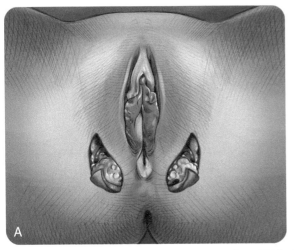 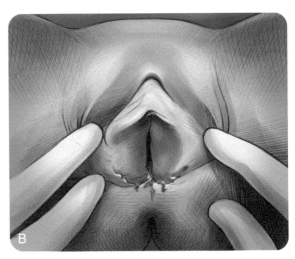

Fig. 4.4 Vulvar stenosis type B, double-perineal-island flaps. (A) Island flaps ready to be tunneled. (B) Island flaps placed to improve stenosis.

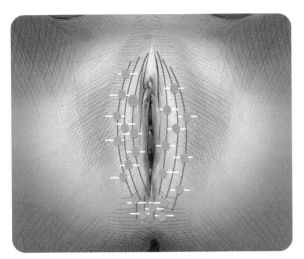 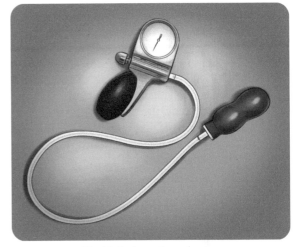

Fig. 4.5 Vulvar stenosis type C as a result of lichen sclerosis: rigotomies and microfat graft.

Fig. 4.6 Postoperative expansion.

VAGINAL VAULT SCAR AFTER VAGINAL HYSTERECTOMY

INDICATIONS: Stable vaginal pain after vaginal vault fixation to sacrospinal ligament nonresponsive to conventional treatments.

SURGICAL STRATEGY:
- HOSPITALIZATION: day surgery
- ANESTHESIA: local + sedation
- ARMAMENTARIUM: microfat graft kit, 21-gauge spinal needle for rigotomies (percutaneous scar release)

- SURGICAL PLAN:
  Trigger points are identified before surgery. Those are two small depressions of the mucosa corresponding to the fixation of the mucosa to the sacrospinus ligament.

  Hydro-dissection with 10 cc of saline + adrenaline 1:100,000 + bupivacaine 2% is injected under the trigger point.

  Three to 5 cc of microfat graft is injected via a 21-gauge spinal needle. The microfat graft can be guided with echography.

The goal of the treatment is to stretch the scar, not to release it completely.

The procedure needs to be repeated 2 to 4 times at 3-month intervals.

- POSTOPERATIVE INDICATIONS: none

TVT MESH EROSION/EXTRUSION

INDICATIONS:

TYPE 1: TVT mesh recurrent erosion of the mucosa

TYPE 2: TVT mesh permanent exposure

SURGICAL STRATEGY:

- HOSPITALIZATION: day surgery
- ANESTHESIA: general or spinal
- ARMAMENTARIUM: microfat graft kit, nanofat graft filtration system, surgical instruments (if needed)
- SURGICAL PLAN:
  - TYPE 1:
    - Day 1 (the day before surgery): The patient is treated with vaginal CO_2 laser, low energy, long pulse, with accurate mapping of the erosions to avoid hitting the exposed mesh. This will determine edema of the mucosa and help to enhance the mucosal thickness that will allow the fat graft.
    - Day 2 (day of surgery): Mucosal microfat graft + nanofat graft of entire vaginal mucosa is performed.
  - TYPE 2:
    - Day 1 (the day before surgery): The patient is treated with vaginal CO_2 laser with accurate mapping of the erosions to avoid hitting the exposed mesh. This will determine edema of the mucosa and help to enhance the mucosal thickness that will allow the fat graft.
    - Day 2 (day of surgery): Removal of the exposed mesh + mucosal microfat graft + nanofat graft of entire vaginal mucosa is performed.

The fat grafting procedure will be repeated 3 times at 3–4-month intervals.

- POSTOPERATIVE INDICATIONS: The pH balance as well as microbiota will be checked periodically.

Expert Profile

Massimiliano Brambilla
Plastic Surgeon
Milan, Italy
Board Certified Plastic Surgeon
Plastic Surgery Service
Department for the Health of the Woman, Child and Newborn
IRCCS Fondazione Cà Granda Ospedale Maggiore Policlinico
Born in 1967 in Milan (Italy).
In 1992, graduated cum laude at the University of Milan with a degree thesis on children intersexual surgery
In 1998, graduated in Plastic Surgery cum laude at the University of Pavia with training in Israel and the United States
Since 1998, has been a surgeon in the Plastic Surgery Division of the IRCCS Fondazione Cà Granda Ospedale Maggiore in Milan, a public institution
In charge of the Services of Genital Plastic Surgery and Breast Plastic Surgery of the Breast Unit
Member of SICPRE and in charge of the SICPRE Genital Chapter
Member of ISPRES, ISAPS, EUSOMA, ASPS, EUGA, ISRAIT, GRIRG
Author of several publications and co-author of 12 books

BIBLIOGRAPHY

Boero V, Brambilla M, Sipio E, et al: Vulvar lichen sclerosus: a new regenerative approach through fat grafting, *Gynecol Oncol* 139:471–475, 2015

Brambilla M: Fat graft of the genital area. In Coleman S, Mazzola R, Pee L, editors: *Fat Injection: From Filling to Regeneration*, 2nd ed., New York, 2017, Thieme [chapter 47].

Brambilla M. Lecture at EUGA (European Society of Urogynecology) meeting, Milan, 21 October 2018.

Brambilla M. Lecture at EUGA (European Society of Urogynecology) meeting, Tel Aviv, 16 October 2019.

Brambilla M. Lecture at EUROGYN meeting, Monaco, 16 November 2018.

Ulrich D, Ulrich F, van Doorn, et al: Lipofilling of perineal and vaginal scars: a new method for improvement of pain after episiotomy and perineal laceration, *Plast Reconstr Surg.* 129: 593e–594e, 2012.

Chapter 5

Hoodplasty

Lina Triana
Plastic Surgeon, Cali, Colombia

Chapter Outline

Expert Approach: Hoodplasty
  Why did you decide to do this technique?
  When did you learn it or if it is your own, how did you end up doing it?
  Can this technique be compared to others and why?
  What do you consider to be important landmarks and anatomy to be able to better perform this technique?
  Can you explain to us how you do the assessment on a patient asking for this procedure? Can you give us some guidelines for constructing an assessment chart?
  Can you describe your technique?
  How can we avoid complications?
  Can you summarize your follow-up and patient recommendations?
  Why do you think this technique should be in the armamentarium of any plastic surgeon?
  What tips can you give us to include this procedure in our practice and how to market it?
Expert Profile

Only a few years ago nobody mentioned the term hoodplasty; it did not exist. But thank goodness, today we just cannot conceive of a labiaplasty without also having the option of a hoodplasty. But before we talk more about this procedure, I would like to mention the importance of treating the entire region.

Not liking our genitalia and having an aesthetic genital procedure is no longer something to be ashamed of. Talking about our vagina is not a taboo any more.

Having aesthetic surgery on our genitalia can be simply because we do not like the appearance, which makes us feel uncomfortable when exposed nude to our partner, or can be secondary to functional concerns that can interfere with our day-to-day activities.

These are the reasons patients undergo an aesthetic genital procedure:

They do not like how it looks:

- Labia minora too long
- Excess skin on the clitoral hood that looks like a penis
- Big clitoral gland
- Too bulky labia majora that show with the use of tight clothes
- Too bulky pubic region that shows through clothes
- Empty labia majora
- Wrinkled labia majora that make you look older down there

Interferes with their daily activities:

- Long labia minora that are pushed inside the vagina during sexual intercourse, making it painful
- Long labia minora that pinch when you ride a bike, a horse, etc.
- Long labia minora that ulcerate with exercise
- Excess skin on clitoral hood that facilitates bad odors
- An overexposed clitoral gland

- An underexposed clitoral gland
- Too little cushion on the pubic area that makes it painful during sexual intercourse

Questions of what is normal in female genital still arise. Many still ask why do surgery in this area? When I listen to these questions, I always think to myself they are being short-sighted. We cannot and must not speak of what is normal in the genital area; every woman is different not only anatomically, but also as to how they perceive their vagina. This is why this procedure, just like any other aesthetic procedure, must be approached in a unique way for each individual patient.

When a labiaplasty is compared with a genital amputation, there is a total misunderstanding of why the procedure is being done. According to the World Heath Organization, a genital amputation is done to limit the woman's sexual life and decrease enjoyment of her sexuality. By performing a genital aesthetic procedure, what is being done is totally the opposite. When performing any of these aesthetic procedures, we are improving the patient's quality of life and how she perceives her genital area.

Also, the phrase "they do not know what else to invent," or "it is just not enough for them to have liposuction and breast augmentation, now they also need to have a procedure done on their genitalia" is synonymous with a person who definitely has not understood the procedure and how important it can be to make one complete. Today, woman are leaders in their families and are also gaining leadership in their jobs. They can be seen as very successful, but still in their sexuality, when they are not comfortable with their genitalia, this can make them feel insecure and prevent them from taking the lead in their intimacy.

Actually, if we only take one thing from this whole chapter, it must be that genital aesthetics is much more than just doing a labiaplasty. When thinking of genital a esthetics, we need to know it is not just one procedure but a group of procedures that will enhance the area.

Also, today we need to know that we can approach the area with surgical and nonsurgical options and this is why it is so important to listen to the patient and understand why she is here with you, asking for an a esthetic genital procedure. This is the only way we can do a correct assessment of the area and end up with the correct treatment plan to be able to have a happy patient.

Surgical aesthetic genital procedures
- Labiaplasty
- Hoodplasty
- Labia majoraplasty
- Hymenoplasty
- Mons pubis plasty

When talking about the external genital aesthetic surgical procedures, we can decrease labia minora size when they are excessive. Here it is important to understand that labia minora are there for a reason and just cutting them all is not the right approach, because it can bring future problems to the patient, such as an open external introitus and/or a dry vagina. When a labiaplasty is performed on a young woman and labia are cut excessively, usually complications will arise when the woman ages, not while they are young and beautiful. This is why it is very important to talk to the patients and explain why you need to leave some labia minora in the area.

A hoodplasty many times can be done as a complementary procedure to a labiaplasty; it can be done alone or as a secondary procedure when during the initial labiaplasty, this area has been ignored.

Labia majoraplasty can be done to remove excess subcutaneous or fatty tissue. That usually includes also taking away excess on the mons pubis region by liposuction or direct excision. Alternatively, in other patients, the approach can be just the opposite: to increase volume in the labia majora and/or the mons pubis region, usually with fat lipoinjection.

Resection of excess skin on the labia majora can also be done and here it is also important not to take too much skin in patients with excessive looseness on the inner thigh region, or those who have a vagina that is too wide. Taking too much labia majora skin in these patients may result in them ending up with an exposed introitus, which is very difficult to correct afterwards. Also, another key aspect to prevent ending up with an exposed introitus is to never plan the inner border resection of the labia majora into the crease that divides the labia minora and majora or beyond the inner hair line of the labia majora. In patients with dark genital skin, it is important to let them know that a labia majora resection scar can be noticeable.

When the mons pubis is ptotic, lifting of the area can also be done and it is important to calculate the lift well, because when done excessively, it can leave the patient with an exposed clitoral gland that might not be appealing, or worse, that can really bother her when wearing tight clothes.

When a hymenoplasty is required in a patient, it is important to explain that this procedure will only cover the vagina entrance and that it will not tighten her vagina. A hymenoplasty, although a simple procedure that consists of reviving the carunculae remnants and suturing them back together, has a high failure rate. I recommend attempting to do a hymenoplasty only in those patients who have these carunculae remnants and not in those whose carunculae are atrophic.

Nonsurgical aesthetic genital procedures:
- G-spot enhancers
- Labia majora-enhancing procedures

Labia majora-enhancing procedures can go from using skin-tightening devices such as radiofrequency and lasers to filling the labia majora with hyaluronic acid. Also, skin lightening procedures with depigmentation creams and lasers can be done in this region.

And with G-spot enhancer procedures, it is very important to explain to the patient that these procedures will only expand the area where more sensitivity receptors are located in the anterior vagina wall. If the patient has a loose vagina, they will not work well, since to have sexual gratification with penetration, there is a need to tighten the vagina during sexual intercourse so that the area with more sensitivity receptors, the anterior vagina wall, is impacted. Also, a G-spot enhancer procedure will not change the maximum erogenous zone of that woman. A G-spot enhancer procedure will simply make this woman feel more when she experiences friction on her anterior vagina wall. The G spot, which is more a zone than a spot, is located in the outer anterior vaginal wall behind and up the pubic bone and can be enhanced by applying hyaluronic acid or platelet-rich plasma in the area.

Expert Approach: Hoodplasty

Lina Triana
Plastic Surgeon
Cali, Colombia

WHY DID YOU DECIDE TO DO THIS TECHNIQUE?

Being a female plastic surgeon, having exposure to aesthetic female patients and giving them the space to really express their concerns gave me the advantage to find out that many of them were uncomfortable with their genital area and just did not know how to express it, or to whom.

This is how I started to become interested in the area to really fulfill these patients' needs. When researching how to do this better, I mostly found techniques on how to reduce labia minora size, not much more.

WHEN DID YOU LEARN IT OR IF IT IS YOUR OWN, HOW DID YOU END UP DOING IT?

I started performing labiaplasties back in 2005 by looking at what could be found in the literature but with a particular interest in not just cutting the excess, since I was just not happy with some of my personal cases. I was not really fulfilling what my patients wanted.

I had two main problems:
1. I could not find the right resection technique.
   - I had patients who just did not like the dark color in their labia minora and when performing the described Alter's wedge technique, this dark color was not going away.
   - Performing the edge resection technique took away the dark skin color, but it was easier to end up with a too short labia minora and/or a showing scar.
2. There was something missing in the overall aesthetics, something even after performing the labiaplasty that made some patients (not all) even unhappier. Why was this happening?

By really observing and listening to my patients, I finally started to understand that what made the difference was whether the patient had excess skin on their clitoral hood or not.

Those patients who had a labiaplasty procedure and had no excess on their clitoral hood were happier, so if the problem was arising when there was an excess on this clitoral hood, how could I correct it?

With the wedge resection, I just could not figure out how to correct large excesses. I even worsened their appearance in the attempt to correct it, but I just did not know why. It took me some time to realize that by resecting the wedge, I was lowering the clitoris hood insertion in the labia minora and that worsened the overall appearance. So how I could prevent this from happening? I needed to find a way to relocate the clitoral hood insertion in the labia minora and could not figure out how to do it with the wedge resection.

This is why I started migrating to the edge resection technique and then incorporated the longitudinal resection of the clitoral hood to finally end up joining both incisions, and by doing so, being able to relocate the insertion of the clitoral hood into the labia minora wherever I wanted.

In 2007, my journey to empower women with their sexual wellbeing through aesthetic plastic surgery procedures began, and with it the sharing of what I have discovered regarding the clitoral hood.

CAN THIS TECHNIQUE BE COMPARED TO OTHERS AND WHY?

Although we call this a hoodplasty procedure, in the end, it is not just "one technique fits all." It all started with the longitudinal resection followed by the edge labia minora resection, but today, there are many other ways to resect based on this initial principle that I will share with you.

WHAT DO YOU CONSIDER TO BE IMPORTANT LANDMARKS AND ANATOMY TO BE ABLE TO BETTER PERFORM THIS TECHNIQUE?

To better perform a hoodplasty, it is very important to locate and mark, before we cut or infiltrate the patient, the insertion of the clitoral hood on the labia minora, which is usually not symmetrical, as well as the frenulum.

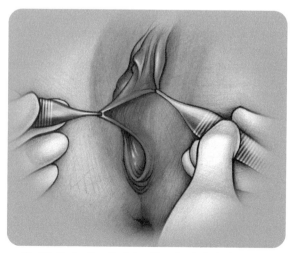

Fig. 5.1 Finding the clitoris hood insertion in the labia minora.

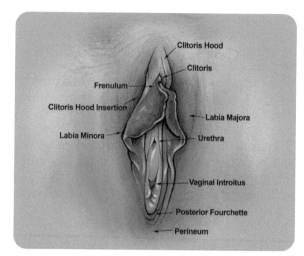

Fig. 5.2 Important anatomical landmark: clitoris hood insertion and frenulum.

Other important anatomical landmarks are the clitoral hood itself, the clitoris gland, and most important the frenulum. Usually the new insertion of the clitoris hood will be relocated upward for a more aesthetic look, near to the patient's frenulum.

CAN YOU EXPLAIN TO US HOW YOU DO THE ASSESSMENT ON A PATIENT ASKING FOR THIS PROCEDURE? CAN YOU GIVE US SOME GUIDELINES FOR CONSTRUCTING AN ASSESSMENT CHART?

There are four types of patients that you will have when offering these types of procedures.

The first patient is one who wants a resection of the labia minora but does not need any work on their clitoral hood. They may have read about the hoodplasty procedure and want to have it done, but just do not need it. In these patients, it is our job as scientific experts to explain why the patient just does not need the procedure.

The second patient comes for a labiaplasty and also needs a hoodplasty to have the best aesthetic result.

The third patient is one who had a labiaplasty done elsewhere and no correction of the clitoral hood was done. This patient unfortunately ends up being more frustrated with her genital appearance after the labiaplasty, since now she looks as if she has a penis down there.

The fourth patient comes with an overexposed clitoris gland that she simply does not like or that is very uncomfortable when friction occurs in the area, for example, when wearing tight clothes.

This exposed clitoral gland can happen because:
She was born like that.

She had a procedure done and too much horizontal resection of the clitoral hood was done.

She takes or took hormone replacement treatments generally recommended in the gym to help body definition. Hormone intake, especially testosterone, can certainly improve our muscle tone and definition and even gets rid of cellulite, but hormone intake can also increase the clitoris length and width, many times making it show too much and look like a real penis. Even worse, is that once these changes occur in the clitoris, they are irreversible; the clitoris will never go back to its normal state.

After identifying whether the patient needs a hoodplasty or not, now you are ready to do the correct assessment of the area:

Does the patient have excess mucosa or a big clitoris?

If there is a big clitoris, I personally do not recommend cutting the clitoral body. I prefer to use a distal horseshoe approach incision and plicate the clitoral body to shorten it. No treatment is available for thinning the clitoral gland or body.

If there is excess clitoral hood, these will be the treatment options:

Longitudinal – Good candidate for a longitudinal resection

Horizontal – Good candidate for a horseshoe resection

CAN YOU DESCRIBE YOUR TECHNIQUE?

There are three main options for this technique:
1. **Longitudinal resection**

    Using a straight forceps, excess skin is clamped; before clamping it, you can find how much excess skin there is by using a similar maneuver to the one we use when doing a pinch blepharoplasty.

    If you are going to do both a labiaplasty and hoodplasty, always start with the hoodplasty, then do the edge resection of the labiaplasty and at the end, unite both resection areas.

    To relocate the clitoral hood insertion, make a three-point stitch: one point going through the inner border of the labia minora, another

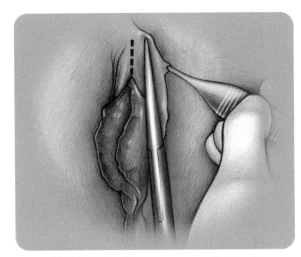

Fig. 5.3 Taking out excess mucosa on clitoral hood.

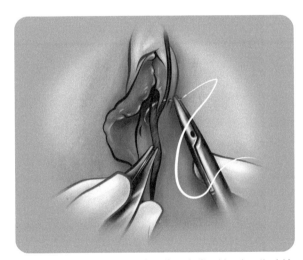

Fig. 5.4 Stitch to relocate new insertion of clitoral hood on the labia minora.

point through the clitoral hood, and the third point through the external border of the labia minora.

    Suturing is done with Vicryl 4-0 running crossed suture for borders eversion.
2. **Horseshoe resection**

    We start with a longitudinal resection that is continued in the midline as a horseshoe resection.
3. **Plication of the clitoral body through a distal horseshoe resection.**

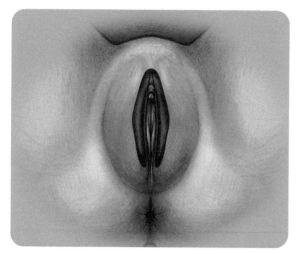

Fig. 5.5 Distal horseshoe resection.

Plication with Vicryl 4-0 is done on each side of the clitoral gland on the horizontal aspect of the clitoral horseshoe resection. When using this plication method, you must always tell the patient that she will experience a little bulky sensation where the plication was done.

HOW CAN WE AVOID COMPLICATIONS?

You can avoid complications by never taking away too much excess on the horizontal horseshoe resection, by never overexposing the clitoral gland, and by taking out the stitches quickly to prevent knots showing.

It is important to explain to the patient that when horseshoe resections are being done, part of the scar is placed on top of the clitoral body and they can feel hard and in some patients be painful when pressure is applied to them.

CAN YOU SUMMARIZE YOUR FOLLOW-UP AND PATIENT RECOMMENDATIONS?

For follow-up, I will take out stitches as early as 6 days after the procedure.
Recommend not wearing tight clothes for 8 days.
100% cotton underwear.
Keep the area dry.
No sexual intercourse or strenuous exercise for 4 weeks (can be less as this area generally heals very quickly).

WHY DO YOU THINK THIS TECHNIQUE SHOULD BE IN THE ARMAMENTARIUM OF ANY PLASTIC SURGEON?

Doing a labiaplasty and not correcting the excess on the clitoral hood when present is something that must be avoided today. Not correcting the excess on the clitoral hood when needed can have a big impact on the patient who in the end feels more unhappy than before having the labiaplasty done. Many times, she believes she just needs to stay like that, as she either does not know there are alternatives for correction of the defect, or simply gives up on seeking them and decides to live like that, more unhappy after having attempted to improve her genital aesthetics. Therefore, if you do not feel comfortable as a surgeon addressing the clitoral hood area with today's knowledge, you should be honest enough with your patient and should not offer labiaplasties. Today, we have the knowledge, training, and experience in the area, so we know that hoodplasty is needed in many patients to fulfill our Hippocratic Oath to always give the best to our patients and never harm them. To honor this oath, if you do not feel comfortable working in this area, you should either not offer labiaplasties, or train yourself in hoodplasties to always offer the best option for the patient.

WHAT TIPS CAN YOU GIVE US TO INCLUDE THIS PROCEDURE IN OUR PRACTICE AND HOW TO MARKET IT?

The best way to include this procedure in your practice is to offer it in all your educational materials to patients, and have the time to really listen to your patient so that she can really open up to you about what bothers her down there. Having it available is not the only key; you need to give them the time to feel confident enough to talk to you about it. Try always to first see the patient dressed so that you can give them the confidence to talk with you about anything and not just see them in a gown and ready to be examined, as this immediately makes the patient feel uncomfortable, preventing her from really expressing herself. Ask her why is she here, and if she mentions something, afterwards, during the exam, give her a mirror so she can see herself and show you what bothers her in her genital region. You can be surprised how what she shows you can be very different from what she told you earlier.

Expert Profile

Lina Triana
Plastic Surgeon
Cali, Colombia

Dr. Lina Triana is a plastic surgeon widely regarded as one of the world's leading experts on the subject of vaginal rejuvenation. Based in Cali, Colombia, Dr. Triana treats patients from all over the world and has been featured in a variety of international media including the BBC. Dr. Lina Triana has been the guest of honor and speaker at more than 50 national and international conferences teaching her colleagues about the latest developments and techniques in vaginal plastic surgery and aesthetic procedures in countries such as Colombia, Venezuela, Peru, Ecuador, Bolivia, Argentina, Chile, Uruguay, Brazil, Mexico, Panama, Guatemala, USA, Canada, France, Monaco, Italy, Belgium, Switzerland, Germany, Greece, Serbia, Turkey, Russia, China, Japan, Vietnam, UAE, Lebanon, Israel, India, Tunisia, Egypt, Saudi Arabia, and South Africa.

Dr. Triana is currently Vice-President of the International Society for Aesthetic Plastic Surgery (ISAPS) and member of its Executive Committee and Board of Directors; Former President and Honorary Member of the Colombian Society of Plastic and Reconstructive Surgery (SCCP); Vice-President and President-Elect 2020–2022 of the Colombian Society of Scientific Societies and member of its Executive Committee and Board of Directors; International member of the American Society for Aesthetic Plastic Surgery (ASAPS), Member of its International and International Fellowship Committees; Member of the International Federation for Plastic Reconstructive and Aesthetic Surgery (FILACP) and member for its Aesthetic Chapter; Honorary Member of the Serbian Society for Plastic, Reconstructive and Aesthetic Surgery (SRBPRAS); Genital Section Editor of ISAPS scientific journal, Aesthetic Plastic Surgery Journal (APS); International Editor of ASAPS scientific journal, the Aesthetic Surgery Journal (ASJ); also, has given multiple scientific inputs to aesthetic plastic surgery while writing book chapters and scientific articles for important scientific journals of aesthetic plastic surgery.

Academic degrees: Doctor and Surgeon, Universidad del Valle, Cali, Colombia. Plastic Reconstructive, Maxillofacial and Hand Surgery, Cirugía Plástica, Universidad del Valle, Cali, Colombia. Age Management, Cenegenics Medical Institute, USA. Aesthetic Plastic Surgery, Clínica Interplástica y Clínica Ivo Pintanguy, Rio di Janeiro, Brazil. Aesthetic Medicine, Universidad de Bolivar, Barranquilla, Colombia. Vaginal Rejuvenation and Design, Laser Vaginal Rejuvenation Institute of America, Dr. David Matlock, Los Ángeles, USA.

BIBLIOGRAPHY

Triana L, Robledo AM: Refreshing labioplasty techniques for plastic surgeons, *Aesthetic Plast Surg.* 36:1078–1086, 2012.
Triana L: *Aesthetic Vaginal Plastic Surgery*, Springer, 2019.
Triana L, Robledo AM: Aesthetic surgery of female external genitalia, *Aesthet Surg J.* 35:165–177, 2015.

Chapter 6

Tightening Inside the Vagina

Lina Triana

Plastic Surgeon, Cali, Colombia

Chapter Outline

Expert Approach: Tightening Inside the Vagina

  Why did you decide to do this technique? When did you learn it or if it is your own, how did you end up doing it?

  Can this technique be compared to others and why?

  What do you consider to be important landmarks and anatomy to be able to better perform this technique?

  Can you explain to us how you do the assessment on a patient asking for this procedure? Can you give us some guidelines for constructing an assessment chart?

  Can you describe your technique?

  How can we avoid complications?

  Can you summarize your follow-up and patient recommendations?

  Why do you think this technique should be in the armamentarium of any plastic surgeon?

  What tips can you give us to include this procedure in our practice and how to market it?

Expert Profile

Today women are not only more aware of their genitalia, but also participate actively in their sexual wellbeing. The concept that the main purpose of sex is for procreation is in the past. Along with the joy of childbirth and kids, woman experience changes in their vagina making it less tight, changes that impact sexual gratification, but woman were silent about it, talking about their sexuality was a tabu.

Why do these vaginal changes happen? With pregnancy, the baby is in the abdomen for approximately 9 months, during which time the weight of this baby is supported by the pelvic floor muscles. After the baby is born, these muscles are elongated after supporting the baby's weight for all this time. As these muscles also support the vagina, after the baby is born, the vagina ends up being loose too.

Having a loose vagina has direct consequences on sexuality because for women, to experience sexual gratification with penetration, they need to feel friction on the anterior vaginal wall. However, if the vaginal walls are loose, they will not be able to contract them as hard as they did before having the baby. Vaginal walls will usually end up being loose during sexual intercourse once the pregnancy ends and the baby is born, but this does not mean that every woman needs a vaginal tightening procedure after childbirth, even though there is certainly some abdominal muscle diastasis.

This situation of feeling less sexual gratification during sexual intercourse is often discounted with the dedication the mother puts into raising her child, plus her busy career agenda, making her unconsciously leaving her sex life on standby, claiming that for her it is not a priority right now, as she has more important things to deal with. Although she initially thinks this is only a transitional period, it can end up staying like this forever, and when the kids are grown, there are fewer and fewer things in common between the couple and in the end, the relationship, as simple as this, can end up having an unhappy ending.

Today we have a more open-minded society where woman not only lead at home, but have leading positions in their careers, giving them the confidence to speak up about their sex life and empower them to have control over seeking ways to improve it.

According to world statistics in 2019 from the International Society of Aesthetic Plastic Surgery, the increase in vaginal rejuvenation procedures is increasing year after year to the point where this is the procedure that has increased the most compared with any other for the last 3 years in a row. For 3 years, two thirds of the total increase in surgical aesthetic procedures was as a result of vaginal rejuvenation procedures.

Now, as plastic surgeons, we are doing more and more labiaplasties. Actually, we are coming to the point that although vaginal rejuvenation is still the procedure that has increased the most compared with all other aesthetic plastic surgery procedures in this past year (2019; 24% increase), and we still have an increase in external vaginal rejuvenation procedures (1% increase of the total 24% increase), now the significant increase comes from vaginal tightening procedures (23% increase of the total 24% increase).

So, the question is, are you doing vaginal plastic surgery procedures in your practice? And if so, what are you doing?

I can now say I have accomplished my goal of making the plastic surgery community understand that vaginal rejuvenation is more than just doing a labiaplasty, but I still need to spread the message that vaginal tightening is not just tightening the vaginal entrance.

After years and years of teaching the concept of vaginal rejuvenation, I can say that in every main scientific meeting, we now have a panel dedicated to vaginal rejuvenation, and now we understand the concept that genital aesthetics is not just cutting the labia minora; it is a group of procedures that enhance the genital area. However, we still need more plastic surgeons doing vaginal tightening procedures, and doing them right.

What do we mean by "doing a vaginal tightening procedure right"? First, we need to remember how woman experience sexual gratification.

There are major differences between males and females regarding genital anatomy and also in how we feel sexual arousal and gratification. Women have several erogenous zones, many even unrelated to direct genital organs. Men have most of their arousal points around the genitalia and more specifically related to friction on the penis. When referring to sexual gratification secondary to sexual intercourse for men, it is much simpler; they need friction on the penis. But for women to have sexual gratification with penetration, they need friction on the anterior vagina wall.

Pregnancies, changes in body weight, or anything that makes the vagina wall less toned will affect sexual gratification for women. During sexual intercourse by penetration, women with loose vaginas are not be able to push the penis toward the anterior vagina wall as hard as before, and as a consequence, less friction in this area, where more sensitivity receptors are present, will happen. If the vagina walls are loose, women cannot contract their vagina walls as hard as before and thus experience less sexual gratification.

Understanding this is crucial for a successful surgery plan. If we think we only need to tighten the entrance of the vagina to increase sexual gratification, we are destined to fail in this procedure and have unhappy patients. The sad part of the story is that many patients will seek a vaginal tightening procedure and if only the entrance is tightened and they still do not have any improvement after the procedure, they can end up thinking that this is the way it has to be, that they will never enjoy their sex life again as when they were younger, and that this is their destiny as women. Do we want this for our patients? Remember once more our Hippocratic Oath: Always give the best to our patients and never harm them. Today, we have the knowledge, so why are we waiting to use the correct approach for vaginal tightening procedures?

Here I also want to add another important concept. Many times, our attention as surgeons is focused on tightening the vagina as much as we can, and this is also the wrong approach. Tightening only the entrance will give sexual satisfaction after the procedure to the partner but not to the patient, and when too much tightening is done, instead of giving any benefit for her, it can even be worse, because having a very tight vagina can be painful for the woman, facilitating tearing of the vaginal wall and ruining her sex life, ending with totally the opposite result of what was intended for the procedure.

Expert Approach: Tightening Inside the Vagina

Lina Triana
Plastic Surgeon
Cali, Colombia

WHY DID YOU DECIDE TO DO THIS TECHNIQUE? WHEN DID YOU LEARN IT OR IF IT IS YOUR OWN, HOW DID YOU END UP DOING IT?

Once I finished my plastic surgery training, I joined a very busy aesthetic plastic surgery practice of three mature male plastic surgeons and my task in the practice was mainly to listen to the patients. I had to do the follow-ups, and in particular, with those who were not happy. I learned that the best thing I could ever do for these patients was to listen to them.

Many times, they had chosen to have the procedure done for the wrong reason, and of course this was the main reason why they were still not happy after having it done. Letting them speak and really listening to them without any judgment was crucial for allowing them to open their hearts to me and show me they were just not happy with their life as a couple. Many wanted to regain their sex lives and were just seeking this with the wrong approach. This is how I became interested in the procedure and started gathering information, first obtaining the knowledge on how to do it, then seeking training, which I did with gynecologists who showed me that tightening the entrance or a little bit of the posterior wall was enough, and lastly, gaining experience on what was best for the patient. After doing the procedure and listening to my patients, I started to discover that just tightening the entrance was not enough to really improve their sexual gratification.

CAN THIS TECHNIQUE BE COMPARED TO OTHERS AND WHY?

Certainly, this technique is similar to when a small prolapse of the posterior or anterior vaginal wall is repaired. It is just the concept of when to do it that makes the difference.

Also, it is important to know that when working on the anterior vaginal wall, depending on how much we go up on the plication, we can even improve stress urinary incontinence, although here we are getting out of our competency zone, so this procedure must never be intended to be done for correction of stress urinary incontinence symptoms. The purpose of the procedure must always be to increase sexual gratification, but often, if the patient also has these symptoms, they will be resolved after the surgery.

WHAT DO YOU CONSIDER TO BE IMPORTANT LANDMARKS AND ANATOMY TO BE ABLE TO BETTER PERFORM THIS TECHNIQUE?

It is important to know that when working on the vaginal cavity, we are working in a corridor-like structure that has distinctive layers such as the mucosa, fascia, and vaginalis muscularis, which are only millimeters wide, and that we are also working very near, only millimeters away, from important pelvic organs, such as the bladder and urethra anteriorly and the rectum posteriorly.

A question that I am constantly asked when training is whether if I do an anterior vaginal wall plication and end up resecting some mucosa, can I damage the G spot/zone. The answer is no, because the G area is up and behind the symphysis bone, very near the vaginal entrance, and the plication does not go that far. However, if we plicate too much in this area, we can end up changing the urovesicular angle, making the patient experience problems during urination.

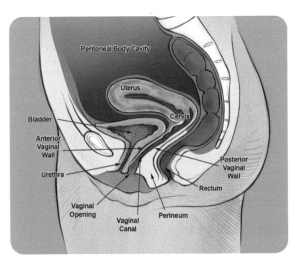

Fig. 6.1 The vagina in proximity to other pelvic organs.

CAN YOU EXPLAIN TO US HOW YOU DO THE ASSESSMENT ON A PATIENT ASKING FOR THIS PROCEDURE? CAN YOU GIVE US SOME GUIDELINES FOR CONSTRUCTING AN ASSESSMENT CHART?

It is important always to first ask why they are there. You really need to understand the reason why they are seeking the procedure. It is also important to ask about stress urinary symptoms and questions about vaginal lubrication.

We have already mentioned that a vaginal tightening procedure is not intended to solve any urinary stress incontinence symptoms, but many times it will resolve them. However, if prolapses are found, the patient should be redirected to another specialist.

Then you need to do an internal vaginal exam. You start the exam by asking the patient to push and actively look for any prolapses. Then you need to touch and feel the vaginal entrance and the inner vaginal walls to properly plan the procedure. How much you are going to do depends on how and where you feel the need to improve the vaginal tone. If you feel the vaginal anterior wall is loose, you will do an anterior vaginoplasty; if the posterior wall is loose, you will do a posterior vaginoplasty; and if the entrance is loose, you will do a perineoplasty. You do not need to do all three procedures in all patients; it will depend on how and where you feel the loss in vaginal tone as to where you will focus your repair. However, it is very common that the patient needs all three repairs.

It is also important to tell the patient that if she suffers from vaginal dryness, this will not be fixed with the procedure, and that if she lubricates too much during sexual intercourse, that cannot be solved either.

CAN YOU DESCRIBE YOUR TECHNIQUE?

Once you do the correct surgery plan for a vaginal tightening procedure based on your assessment, if all three approaches are needed (an anterior and posterior vaginoplasty plus a perineoplasty), you will start with the anterior vaginoplasty first, then move to mark and take away the excess mucosa on the perineal areas, continue with the posterior vaginoplasty, and finish with the muscle repair and mucosa closure of the perineoplasty.

Starting with the Posterior Vaginoplasty

An internal pudendal block is done.

A labia majora retractor is used.

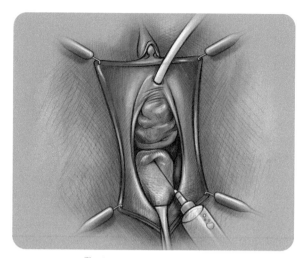

Fig. 6.2 Anterior hydro-dissection.

Infiltration is done with saline solution and adrenaline on the anterior and posterior vaginal walls.

The uterus, cervix, or vaginal cupula (if the patient has previously undergone a hysterectomy) are pulled down.

A horizontal incision is done at the midline on the anterior vaginal wall, approximately 2 cm from the cervix neck.

Dissection of the mucosa is done starting from the cervix to the urethra along the midline. The use of a tentlike dissection, with one Allis forceps being distal to the dissection point and two other Allis forceps,

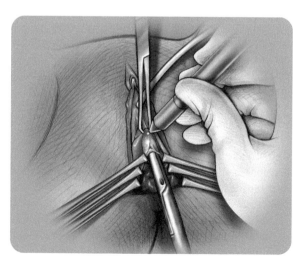

Fig. 6.3 Flap elevation.

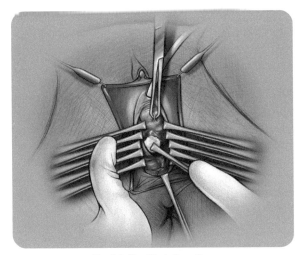

Fig. 6.4 Flap blunt dissection.

one on each side of the horizontal incision borders, is done, prolonging the incision upwards until a change from smooth to rough mucosa is seen. Another way of finding out where to stop the upward dissection is to pull the urine catheter and feel its balloon. This is the urovesical angle and the dissection should never go beyond this point to prevent further urinary complications.

Blunt lateral dissection is done, exposing loose fascia, and hemostasis is done.

Plication of the fascia starting from the urethra towards the cervix is done from lateral border to lateral border, avoiding the suture passing through the

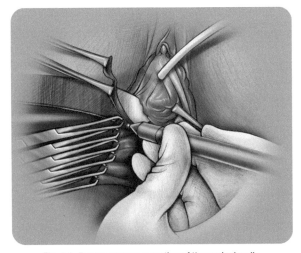

Fig. 6.5 Excess mucosa resection of the vaginal walls.

midline. Remember, here it is easy to compromise the urethra, which is only centimeters away from the area where we are working. To facilitate suturing, you need to hold the needle holder and needle at a different angle than that generally used to suture skin. Suturing is done with Vicryl 2-0 in a two-layer manner, first a running locked suture and then a second layer with single crossed sutures, just like we do on an abdominal fascia tummy tuck plication. Excess mucosa is trimmed on each side.

Mucosa borders are sutured with Vicryl 2-0 running locked sutures, starting from the urethra to the cervix.

Perineoplasty Markings

The midline is marked at the perineal region making sure it is several millimeters above the anal mucocutaneous junction. Making this marking above the anal mucocutaneous junction makes you, the surgeon, stay away from the anal sphincter, once resecting the excess perineal skin. Excess skin to be resected at the perineal mucosa borders is calculated by approximating two mosquito forceps at the midline, defining the new size of the external introitus and making sure the internal introitus (where the carunculae remnants are) never end up being smaller than the external introitus.

Excess perineal mucosa is elevated.

Posterior Vaginoplasty

Dissection of perineal skin is continued inside the posterior vaginal wall from the vaginal entrance towards the cervix in the same way as it was done on the anterior vaginal wall. It can be helpful to pull the uterus up to facilitate dissection secondary to tension.

Dissection of the lateral flaps is also done as in the anterior vaginoplasty.

Fascia plication in a running locked suture is done and a second suture layer is done the same as in the anterior fascia plication. This is done from the cervix towards the internal introitus, where it is stopped.

Suturing of the posterior vaginal mucosa is done from the cervix to the internal introitus.

Finishing with the Perineoplasty

The pubococcygeal muscle borders are approximated in the middle with several Vicryl 2-0 sutures, at least three.

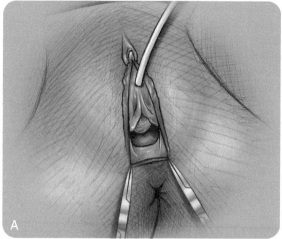

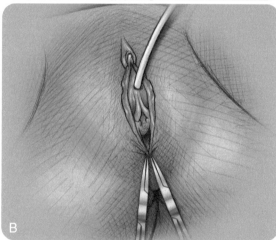

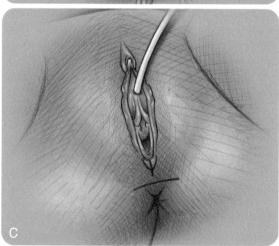

Fig. 6.6 Excess perineal mucosa. (A) Two mosquito forceps. (B) Mosquito forceps brought to the midline. (C) Excess perineal mucosa marked.

Approximation of the labia minora skin is done with Vicryl 2-0 and then the rest of the mucosa is sutured from the internal to the external introitus and also the perineal mucosa, all done with the same Vicryl 2-0.

HOW CAN WE AVOID COMPLICATIONS?

Infiltration with saline solution and adrenaline is a crucial step that should be done before starting any cutting. This infiltration not only decreases bleeding but more importantly, gives a hydro-dissection effect.

It is very important to always be aware during the mucosa elevation that you are only millimeters from important pelvic organs.

Also, on the anterior fascia plication, avoid the midline to prevent pinching the urethra. It is advisable to prevent pinching other structures to always introduce the needle placating the fascia on the lateral aspects of the plication and never on the midline.

And NEVER leave an inner introitus smaller than the outer introitus. It will lead to trauma and tearing of the vaginal entrance with penetration.

CAN YOU SUMMARIZE YOUR FOLLOW-UP AND PATIENT RECOMMENDATIONS?

Eight days of no tight clothing and 100% cotton underwear is recommended.

No sexual intercourse or exercising for 6 weeks.

Antiseptic baths in the area for the first 3 days after the procedure.

WHY DO YOU THINK THIS TECHNIQUE SHOULD BE IN THE ARMAMENTARIUM OF ANY PLASTIC SURGEON?

Not only is this technique a must in the plastic surgeon's armamentarium because it is a procedure that is highly in demand these days, but also because it can really empower women. Today, women are leaders in their families and in their jobs, and giving them the option of also leading in their sex lives really empowers them, makes them complete.

Also, it is very important that we plastic surgeons embrace vaginal tightening surgical procedures. We must never forget successful outcomes, for example, what happened when liposuction was first described. We were not sure if it was the right thing for our patients, if it was safe, if we should do it as plastic surgeons. Thank goodness we evolved in the right direction. We embraced liposuction and today, it is one of the most popular procedures that we plastic surgeons do. The same must happen with vaginal tightening surgical approaches. If we do not start doing the procedure now, if we send the patients to other specialists, we are at risk of losing these patients and repeating what happened several years ago when our patients wanted nonsurgical options and we as surgeons sent them to other doctors because as surgeons, we were supposed only to do surgery. As a result, these patients started to build trust in these nonplastic surgeons and ended up having aesthetic procedures, even plastic surgeries, with these noncore doctors. Today, we share facial aesthetic surgery; do we want to do the same with body contouring? The future of our specialty is in our hands, we need to train ourselves in vaginal aesthetic plastic surgery.

WHAT TIPS CAN YOU GIVE US TO INCLUDE THIS PROCEDURE IN OUR PRACTICE AND HOW TO MARKET IT?

A good starting point to introduce the procedure is have it in your educational material and also find a mechanism to ask the patient about urinary stress incontinence. These symptoms can be the door, so the patient can feel free to discuss with us if she wants to improve something regarding her loose vagina.

Expert Profile

Lina Triana
Plastic Surgeon
Cali, Colombia

Dr. Lina Triana is a plastic surgeon widely regarded as one of the world's leading experts on the subject of vaginal rejuvenation. Based in Cali, Colombia, Dr. Triana treats patients from all over the world and has been featured in a variety of international media, including the BBC. Dr. Triana has been the guest of honor and speaker at more than 50 national and international conferences, teaching her colleagues about the latest developments and techniques in vaginal plastic surgery and aesthetic procedures in Colombia, Venezuela, Peru, Ecuador, Bolivia, Argentina, Chile, Uruguay, Brazil, Mexico, Panama, Guatemala, United States, Canada, France, Monaco, Italy, Belgium, Switzerland, Germany, Greece, Serbia, Turkey, Russia, China, Japan, Vietnam, UAE, Lebanon, Israel, India, Tunisia, Egypt, Saudi Arabia, and South Africa.

Dr. Triana is currently vice-president of the International Society for Aesthetic Plastic Surgery (ISAPS) and member of its executive committee and board of directors; former president and honorary member of the Colombian Society of Plastic and Reconstructive Surgery (SCCP); vice-president and president-elect 2020–2022 of the Colombian Society of Scientific Societies and member of its executive committee and board of directors; international member of the American Society for Aesthetic Plastic Surgery (ASAPS), member of its International and International Fellowship Committees; member of the International Federation for Plastic Reconstructive and Aesthetic Surgery (FILACP) and member of its Aesthetic Chapter; honorary member of the Serbian Society for Plastic, Reconstructive and Aesthetic Surgery (SRBPRAS); genital section editor of ISAPS scientific journal, Aesthetic Plastic Surgery Journal (APS); The ASAPS scientific journal is called Aesthetic Surgery Journal (ASJ) International Editor of ASAPS scientific journal, the Aesthetic Surgery Journal (ASJ); also, has given multiple scientific inputs to aesthetic plastic surgery while writing book chapters and scientific articles for important scientific journals of aesthetic plastic surgery.

Academic degrees: Doctor and Surgeon, Universidad del Valle, Cali, Colombia. Plastic Reconstructive, Maxillofacial and Hand Surgery, Cirugía Plástica, Universidad del Valle, Cali, Colombia. Age Management, Cenegenics Medical Institute, USA. Aesthetic Plastic Surgery, Clínica Interplástica y Clínica Ivo Pintanguy, Rio di Janeiro, Brazil. Aesthetic Medicine, Universidad de Bolivar, Barranquilla, Colombia. Vaginal Rejuvenation and Design, Laser Vaginal Rejuvenation Institute of America, Dr. David Matlock, Los Angeles, CA, USA.

BIBLIOGRAPHY

Triana L: Vaginal tightening: surgical and non-surgical options. In Nahai F, editor: *The Art of Aesthetic Surgery: Principles and Techniques*, 3rd ed., St Louis, 2005, Quality Medical Publishing [chapter 100b].
Triana L: *Aesthetic Vaginal Plastic Surgery*, New York, 2019, Springer.

Chapter 7

Scrotal Lift

Introduction Lina Triana Invited Expert

Enzo Citarella, Plastic Surgeon, Cali, Colombia, Rio di Janerio, Brazil

Chapter Outline

Why Offer a Scrotal Lift?

Why It Is Important as Doctors to Offer These Types of Treatments?

Important Anatomy

Other Approaches to the Area

Expert Approach: Scrotal Lift

Why did you decide to do this technique?

When did you learn it or If it is your own, how did you end up doing it?

What do you consider to be important landmarks and anatomy to be able to better perform this technique?

Can you explain to us how you do the assessment on a patient asking for the procedure? Can you give us some guidelines for constructing an assessment chart?

Can you describe your technique?

How can we avoid complications?

Can you summarize your follow-up and patient recommendations?

Why do you think this technique should be in the armamentarium of any plastic surgeon?

What tips can you give us to include this procedure in our practice and how to market it?

Expert Profile

Different Expert Approach: Scrotal Lift

Many might say, why is there a need to lift the scrotal area? Well, just like women lift their breasts, men can also lift their scrotal area.

Because we live on planet Earth and planet Earth has gravity, our bodies are constantly exposed to this downward force that makes everything fall, and and testes are no exception.

Testes are supported in a cutaneous sac for a reason—to protect spermatozoids from dying as a result of high temperatures. The internal average temperature of the body is 42 °C, but thanks to the scrotal sac, the temperature of the testes is a couple of degrees lower.

However, as it is named, it is a "sack" that supports the weight of the testes, and over time it starts to elongate. This, plus the aging process of this naturally thin skin makes it not only ptotic but wrinkled, making it look old.

The situation is even more evident as today, men tend to shave down there, just like women do. As men, they can go to the gym, even help themselves with some hormone replacement to make themselves look younger, so this elongated and wrinkled scrotal sac just does not fit with this masculine body. Also, with hormone use, the penis size can decrease, making the scrotal sac hang and show even more. This is why more and more men are seeking this type of procedure.

Why Offer a Scrotal Lift?

With time everything falls, and the scrotal region is no exception.

Having a masculine, defined body is synonymous with being young and fit, and an elongated and wrinkled scrotal region just does not match this appearance.

Taking hormones, especially to better define their bodies, can have consequences in men, such as a decrease in penis size, making the hanging scrotal region more evident.

Why It Is Important as Doctors to Offer These Types of Treatments?

As we all know, our specialty was born after there was enough technology to save soldiers that were injured in battle, but even though they were saved, they still did not want to live. Therefore, a group of doctors who were more open to listening to their patients understood that it was more important to work towards improving the quality of life of these patients, rather than to save them but leave them with sequelae that did not allow them to experience life in the same way as before they were injured.

So, if we keep on the same line of thinking, aesthetic plastic surgery is no different. We are here to improve the patient's quality of life and if a scrotal lift will help develop confidence in a man who is fighting against aging, why not help him?

Important Anatomy

The scrotum is the skin that continues from the lower abdomen and behind the penis, forming a sac surrounding the testes.

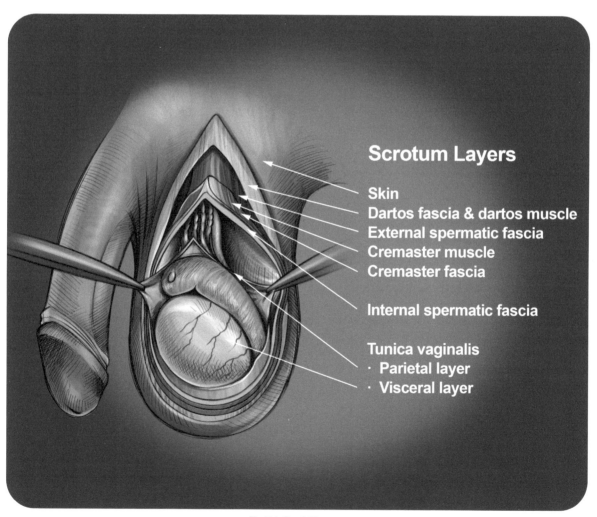

Scrotum Layers

Skin
Dartos fascia & dartos muscle
External spermatic fascia
Cremaster muscle
Cremaster fascia

Internal spermatic fascia

Tunica vaginalis
· Parietal layer
· Visceral layer

Fig. 7.1 Scrotal layers.

The scrotum is made of layers, the skin and the dartos being the most relevant for this scrotal lift procedure.

The dartos or dartos fascia is a layer of connective tissue that surrounds the scrotum and also surrounds the penis, being called in this area the superficial fascia of the penis, and when it extends to the abdomen it becomes Scarpa's fascia.

Dartos fascia is superficial to the spermatic fascia and is important in reducing the temperature of the testes. Dartos fascia contains smooth muscle responsible for the wrinkling and expansion of the scrotal skin used for temperature control of the area. Its innervation comes from the ilioinguinal and posterior scrotal nerves.

Other Approaches to the Area

It is common for us to recommend hydrating creams and lotions when we have wrinkled skin or to even promote the use of these to prevent wrinkles from appearing. However, the scrotal area is exposed to heat and commonly can sweat. When applying lotions or creams, often the skin can tend to sweat more, so using conventional hydrating creams in this area is not recommended.

Also, using different skin-tightening nonsurgical procedures has not been explored yet, perhaps because scrotal skin is very thin and sensitive to heat exposure, and all these skin-tightening technologies are based on energy devices that produce some kind of heat. Remember that testes should not be exposed to high temperatures.

Expert Approach: Scrotal Lift

Enzo Citarella
Plastic Surgeon
Rio di Janeiro, Brazil

Dr. Enzo Rivera Citarella is well known worldwide as a plastic surgeon for facial rejuvenation, and through time, after listening to his patients, has discovered this innovative procedure, being a pioneer in this field of scrotal lift surgery. Let us see what he has to tell us regarding this unique approach to male genital rejuvenation.

WHY DID YOU DECIDE TO DO THIS TECHNIQUE?

I realized that scrotoplasty surgery was not readily available and it was something some of my patients had asked me about, as they were concerned that their testes looked aged compared with the rest of their body after undergoing other cosmetic procedures.

WHEN DID YOU LEARN IT OR IF IT IS YOUR OWN, HOW DID YOU END UP DOING IT?

The urologists, who were the most exposed to these patients' concerns, had not conceived of this surgery. So, after listening to my patients' concerns, I decided I really wanted to help them and started to design the surgery myself.

I thought about doing a horizontal incision and where was best to place it, discussed it with a very experienced urologist I knew, and started putting together the procedure. Also, I realized that careful resection of the skin without compromising underlying structures was necessary to have a successful outcome, and therefore I started performing scrotoplasties. As a general surgeon as well as a plastic surgeon, I knew the anatomy, and this was how I started to do the procedure 5 years ago.

WHAT DO YOU CONSIDER TO BE IMPORTANT LANDMARKS AND ANATOMY TO BE ABLE TO BETTER PERFORM THIS TECHNIQUE?

It is important to identify the dartos fascia as this has to be preserved along with the deeper anatomical structures (external spermatic fascia, cremaster muscle, internal spermatic fascia, and tunica vaginalis). Consequently, just the skin is resected.

CAN YOU EXPLAIN TO US HOW YOU DO THE ASSESSMENT ON A PATIENT ASKING FOR THE PROCEDURE? CAN YOU GIVE US SOME GUIDELINES FOR CONSTRUCTING AN ASSESSMENT CHART?

The patient has to be unhappy with the excess skin on his testes. This is the most important factor. The patient really has to have excess skin so that a resection can be done. After resection, the skin borders surrounding the testes need to be sutured together with just enough tension, but not too much.

The assessment is therefore done at the preoperative stage and is on an individual basis. The amount of skin to be resected varies from patient to patient, and there are no specific landmarks. Some patients have more excess skin than others. The skin to be resected must be measured before starting the scrotoplasty surgery. The patient is marked while in a standing position, and the markings are done based on a pinch test to measure how much skin will be resected. As the scrotal skin is very elastic, you must not be shy on the resection.

CAN YOU DESCRIBE YOUR TECHNIQUE?

A scrotoplasty surgery consists of resecting the excess cutaneous tissue while preserving the dartos fascia and the other deep anatomical structures. The skin is marked with a pinch test; a transverse ellipse is drawn in methylene blue.

Infiltration in the subdermal plane is performed with a vasoconstrictive solution of normal saline with 1:200,000 epinephrine. The incision is performed with a 15 scalpel blade, preserving the dartos fascia and the deeper anatomical planes, while the surgical assistant creates tension on the skin with small hooks and Allis clamps at each end of the markings. The scar is hidden on the posterior aspect of the scrotal sac, behind the testes. Although skin dissection can be extensive, there is little risk of skin necrosis, as this skin is highly vascularized.

The excess skin is excised and rigorous hemostasis is performed. The skin is approximated with absorbable catgut 4-0 sutures in separate "U" stitches,

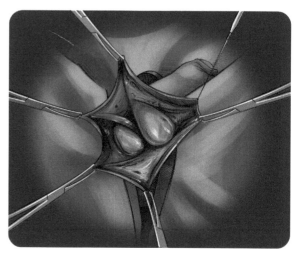

Fig. 7.3 Dissection of just the scrotal skin preserving the deeper anatomical planes.

placing the scar in the posterior–inferior region of the scrotum. An occlusive dressing is placed for 24 h postoperatively.

HOW CAN WE AVOID COMPLICATIONS?

As with all surgical procedures, there are many things that can be done to avoid complications. Making sure the patient is a decent weight (a healthy BMI) and healthy enough to undergo surgery is very important (ensuring that all their preoperative tests are done), ensuring the operating theater has all the necessary resources, putting on an occlusive dressing that will help prevent complications in the first few hours, making sure the patient has regular follow-ups, rests, and does not do any strenuous exercise for at least 3 months after surgery.

CAN YOU SUMMARIZE YOUR FOLLOW-UP AND PATIENT RECOMMENDATIONS?

The patient can go home on the same day of surgery (it is an outpatient procedure) with an occlusive dressing that he will wear for 24 hours. The occlusive dressing consists of gauze and cotton that are held together with an elastic bandage wrapped around the genital area, simulating underwear.

He will be seen again the next day to remove the dressing and ensure that everything is healing well. Four days after the procedure, the patient is seen again, then 1 week after, and at 1 month, 3 months, and 6 months

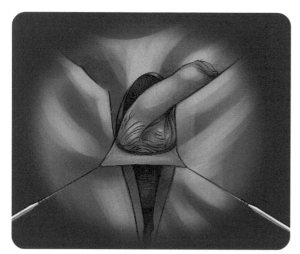

Fig. 7.2 Horizontal incision at the base on the posterior aspect of the scrotal sac.

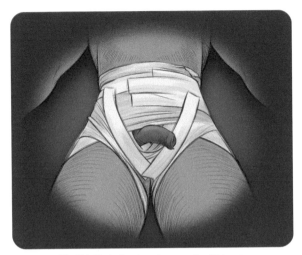

Fig. 7.4 Occlusive dressing worn for 24 hours.

after the procedure. He should rest for the first 2 weeks and should not do strenuous exercise for 3 months.

WHY DO YOU THINK THIS TECHNIQUE SHOULD BE IN THE ARMAMENTARIUM OF ANY PLASTIC SURGEON?

The patients are very happy with the results after surgery, with this procedure having a high level of satisfaction. It is also a simple surgery that takes a relatively short time.

Plastic surgeons who perform, esthetic work should all know how to perform this procedure as a way to rejuvenate the testes. Resecting this excess skin makes men feel young again and it also helps them in functional aspects; it is not a purely aesthetic procedure. Long-hanging testes may get in the way of doing everyday activities such as running, biking, walking, or even sitting or driving. Taking away this hanging weight can also help with lumbar pain, as a sagging scrotum can have a pulling effect, creating strain on the lumbar nerves.

WHAT TIPS CAN YOU GIVE US TO INCLUDE THIS PROCEDURE IN OUR PRACTICE AND HOW TO MARKET IT?

You can market it as "testicular rejuvenation for men" and also emphasize that it is not a purely aesthetic procedure; it also helps in a functional way when the testes start to sag with time and get in the way of day-to-day activities. It is something that more and more younger men are seeking because of the use of anabolic steroids that can cause excess scrotal skin as a side effect. Also, a lot of older men are interested in having it done for aesthetic and functional purposes, as it also helps with sagging testes that get in the way and are an annoying feeling for these men.

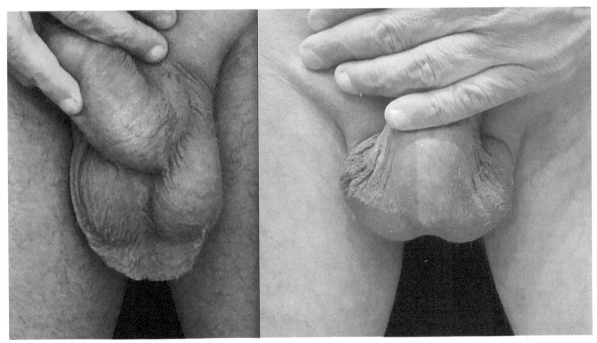

Fig. 7.5 A happy patient who underwent a scrotal lift, which made him feel younger and encouraged him to go to the gym and eat healthily afterwards.

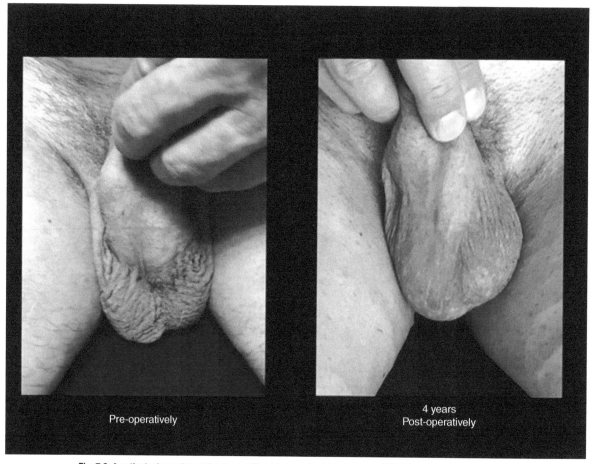

Pre-operatively

4 years
Post-operatively

Fig. 7.6 A patient who underwent a scrotal lift, which resolved his decreased libido and improved his sex life.

All the patients on whom I have performed this surgery are very happy with the results. Plastic surgeons should get testimonials from their patients after performing the scrotoplasty procedure as a source for letting other men know it is a viable option, and of course for marketing purposes. Here are two examples of testimonials from my patients:

"Before surgery, I felt that I was older than my actual age. I was embarrassed to undress in front of others, especially when I would have sexual relations. After the surgery, I feel proud of my body and I feel younger. I have even started a diet to improve my body so it matches the new aesthetics of my testicles."

"I decided to have surgery because the excess skin of my testicles made me feel old and it affected my sex life to the point it would lower my libido; I would even sometimes avoid my partner. I would also feel discomfort when sitting down or driving."

Expert Profile

Enzo José Rivera Citarella
Plastic Surgeon
Rio di Janeiro, Brazil
Graduated in medicine from the Universidad del Norte, Barranquilla, Colombia.

Plastic and reconstructive surgeon of the Ivo Pitanguy Institute in Rio de Janeiro, Brazil (chief resident).

Fellowship in endoscopic plastic surgery with Dr. Nicanor Isse in Burbank, CA, USA.

Appointed by the Municipal Chamber of Rio de Janeiro to the role of Honorary Citizen of the Municipality of Rio de Janeiro.

Member of the Brazilian Plastic Surgery Society (SBCP), participating actively in the society's reunions and committees.

Member of the Colombian Plastic Surgery Society.

Member of ISAPS.

Member of the Ivo Pitanguy Ex-Alumni Association (AEXPI).

Assistant professor, member of staff, and coordinator of the endoscopic department at the Ivo Pitanguy Institute.

Has been a member of the Brazilian Plastic Surgery Society's board of directors for several years.

Member of the International Committee of the Brazilian Plastic Surgery Society, for the Rio de Janeiro region.

Participated in multiple surgical demonstrations in different countries around the world.

Author of the book *Endoscopia da Região Frontal* (Endoscopy of the Frontal Region), which was translated into three languages, and several articles related to endoscopy associated with rhytidectomy surgery.

Author of multiple articles related to the treatment of the mid third of the face and the management of the deep structures of the neck in order to define its contour, which is some evidence of his vast experience.

Different Expert Approach: Scrotal Lift

David Caminer
Plastic Surgeon
Australia

I have performed scrotoplasties for many years and in my opinion, I like to hide the scar in the midline raphe of the scrotum. It is a fairly simple procedure in which once a wedge resection is done in a vertical dimension with a vertical ellipse, one can reduce the scrotum in a transverse and a horizontal position by taking the ellipse further around the inferior surface of the scrotum. I believe this is better than a transverse resection because in a transverse resection, you need to make the incision posteriorly and one can end up with dog ears, which can make the scrotum look a little unusual on each side. The lift other than this is the same in that one excises skin plus underlining dartos muscle, and then does a meticulous repair of the layers.

BIBLIOGRAPHY

Alter GJ: Aesthetic genital surgery. In Neligan PC, Warren P, editors: *Plastic Surgery*, 3rd ed, Philadelphia, 2012, Saunders/Elsevier, pp 1212–1234, *Aesthetic Surgery*, vol. 2.

Armando LJ, Sowerby JS, Kanarogolu N: Preliminary report on a new surgical technique for the management of bothersome scrotomegaly in selected adolescent males, *J Pediatric Urol.* 11:295–298, 2015.

Chapter 8

Penile Enlargement: Suspensory Ligament, Fat Grafting, Scrotal Webbing

Introduction Lina Triana Invited Expert

David Caminer, Plastic Surgeon, Cali, Colombia, Sydney Australia

Chapter Outline

Expert Approach to Penile Enlargement: Suspensory Ligament, Fat Grafting, Scrotal Webbing

Why did you decide to do this technique?

When did you learn it or if it is your own, how did you end up doing it?

Can this technique be compared to others and why?

What do you consider to be important landmarks and anatomy to be able to better perform this technique?

Can you explain to us how do you do the assessment on a patient asking for this procedure? Can you give us some guidelines for constructing an assessment chart?

Can you describe your technique?

How can we avoid complications?

Can you summarize your follow-up and patient recommendations?

Why do you think this technique should be in the armamentarium of any plastic surgeon?

What tips can you give us to include this procedure in our practice and how to market it?

Expert Profile

Just as female genital surgery has been increasing exponentially in the past years, male genital surgery is now becoming more available and with better outcomes, and I am sure that will start increasing also.

Today, more and more men are asking for body definition surgeries and male genital aesthetics serve well to provide a better harmonious figure overall.

Because function is so important, often men were afraid of having these procedures, worrying that in the end they could end up with negative consequences in sexual function, but now we know it is just the opposite. Although the genital aesthetic procedures do not directly improve sexual function in men, from a psychological point of view, feeling more comfortable with their penis length and overall appearance also increases male general confidence.

Penile lengthening procedures as well as increasing the penile girth are generally requested by young adult males who although they do not present with real sexual dysfunction, do feel uncomfortable when referring to their size.

Penile enlargement surgeries can also be included with scrotal procedures for a complete male genital rejuvenation. Just as in women, one must not only talk about one part but the overall male genital aesthetics.

Let's see what our expert has to tell us. Dr. David Caminer has more than 15 years of experience in the field. While thinking outside the box in ways on how to better serve his patients, he came up with these new modifications to previously described techniques to really impact the overall surgical outcomes in male genital surgery.

Expert Approach to Penile Enlargement: Suspensory Ligament, Fat Grafting, Scrotal Webbing

David Caminer
Plastic Surgeon
Sydney, Australia

WHY DID YOU DECIDE TO DO THIS TECHNIQUE?

I have been working on my technique for 20 years. I decided to perform this operation the way that I do it so that the complications that I was seeing from others would be minimized. This technique has evolved over the years so I can tell my patients that there will be minimal bad sequelae as a result of the operation. I was seeing some bad complications and it was ruining people's lives, so I wanted to do a very safe technique.

WHEN DID YOU LEARN IT OR IF IT IS YOUR OWN, HOW DID YOU END UP DOING IT?

I learned part of the technique, the division of the suspensory ligament, from urologists, but that is not the complicated part. The issue and the problems that I was seeing were from the fat grafting into the dead space once the suspensory ligament was divided. I felt that filling the dead space with vascularized fat was better than a thick/large piece of nonvascularized fat graft. Just dividing the ligament and not filling the dead space with tissue meant that the scarring would pull the penis up again and the result would be poor. This is the reason historically why penile lengthening by ligament division alone has a very poor reputation.

When I performed a few of these procedures in the area, I noticed quite a lot of fat laterally. I worked out a way to elevate a distally based fat flap and used one from each side to fill the dead space created by the suspensory ligament division.

The other complication I was seeing was related to degloving the penis and using a dermis fat graft as a wrap around the penile shaft for girth augmentation.

Fat grafting worked well for me in other areas with very few complications, so I started to use fat grafting for girth augmentation.

I have been performing this technique for about 15 years now and have found it to be excellent, with very few complications.

The incision that I perform is for a V–Y advancement flap. This flap has evolved over the last 10 years. At the beginning, I was doing a transverse incision, but I was only getting approximately a maximum of 2 cm increase in length. I was worried about the scar in that area but at some stage, I discussed it with a patient, and he was not worried about the scar if it increased the length gain. I thus decided to do a V–Y advancement flap. The function of this flap is to gain more skin over the proximal penile shaft, which I believe is part of the issue of why penises cannot be extended as much without doing that incision. I have been using this incision in all cases for many years now. I believe that using this V–Y advancement flap incision makes a difference in the final result of the procedure.

CAN THIS TECHNIQUE BE COMPARED TO OTHERS AND WHY?

Yes, this technique can certainly be compared with the other techniques. In all penile lengthening techniques, the suspensory ligament needs to be divided.

How one fills the dead space to keep the penis from retracting back is the difference. This technique can be compared with dermal grafting, but with dermal fat grafting, the problem is with such a big lump of fat, there is often an amount of necrosis that occurs. Whatever necrosis occurs leads to more fibrosis. Fibrosis should be avoided at all costs. Any fibrosis of the penile shaft to the pubis is detrimental for penile length.

The fat flap is a random pedicle vascularized flap. I have not seen any fat necrosis or infection sequelae of these fat flaps. I believe that even in thin people, one can find enough fat tissue in the area to fill this space. Obviously, the fatter the patient is, the more fat there is to harvest. I believe this to be the best scenario. However, if the patient is too fat, his pubic pannus will work against penile length, as it will engulf the penile shaft.

One of the advantages of harvesting fat from the inguinal region and spermatid cord area is that it does make this area less bulky and one can see a flattening of the pubic contour of the area, which many men like.

If people are overweight and need liposuction around the mons pubis area, my recommendation would be that the penile lengthening procedure is performed first. I would not do the liposuction and the penile augmentation at the same time. This is because the area is the most dependent part of the abdomen, leading to prolonged and excessive swelling which delays the healing process. I would stagger the sequence of the liposuction and would recommend that one perform the liposuction at a later stage once the penile lengthening procedure has settled down. I would recommend waiting 4 months before performing liposuction when it is necessary.

My experience with patients who have had liposuction to the pubic area on a prior occasion is that it is usually done on the more central area and does not interfere with the harvesting or the amount of fat that can be harvested from the spermatic cord.

This technique also differs from other techniques of fat grafting of the penile shaft for increased girth.

I am not a fan of dermal fat grafting of the penile shaft. When performing dermal fat grafting of the shaft, one needs to deglove the penis. With any degloving of an organ like this, there is always the possibility of skin necrosis. If, unfortunately, there is a significant amount of skin necrosis in that area, the result is devastating to the patient. I hence stay away from this technique and as such, I think microfat grafting is such a good technique with no chance at all of any skin necrosis of the penile shaft. Other reasons for not liking this technique of dermis fat grafting are the long scars that result from the harvesting of this tissue. There is also the issue of too much bulk at the base of the penis, giving the penis the Eiffel Tower appearance. This is why it is my preferred technique for girth augmentation.

All the articles and myths of lumpiness and no fat take has not been my experience. I harvest the fat as microfat rather than as a normal fat graft with smaller holes in the cannulae. When performing microfat grafting, the contour of the penis is very good and can be adjusted with ease. I do not see any lumpiness.

Fat grafting can be redone if the patient wants further girth increase 6 months after the first procedure.

I do tell the patients they will lose about 50% of the fat. When they wake up, there will have considerable swelling and this does resolve over about 3 weeks. It will take about 4 months to see the final outcome regarding the fat take.

A question that patients often ask is, "Will my penis feel soft?" This does not seem to be a problem. The fat that remains is not such a large amount as to make the penis become soft and boggy. I also believe that with fat grafting, there is certain amount of fibrosis that occurs, and this gives the penis a fairly firm consistency.

WHAT DO YOU CONSIDER TO BE IMPORTANT LANDMARKS AND ANATOMY TO BE ABLE TO BETTER PERFORM THIS TECHNIQUE?

I think a good understanding of the anatomy of the area is essential. The penile anatomy is not that difficult. One needs to understand that there are the dorsal penile nerves, which is one's main concern when dividing the ligament. One should stay out of the Buck's fascia in that area in order to preserve the nerves. This plane is fairly easy to see and to follow down the penile shaft. I dissect as far as the inferior aspect of the pubic symphysis. At this point, the symphysis takes an upward turn, and this is where I stop the dissection. At this point, the neurovascular structures become more at risk of injury.

Other important anatomy is when harvesting the spermatic cord fat flaps, one should understand that any structure in the cord can be divided and understanding the anatomy of the spermatic cord is important. I think the two main structures that worry me are the nerves that travel down in or just adjacent to the cord. I always worry about postoperative long-term pain secondary to nerve injury, as well as numbness. The two nerves in that area are the genital branch of the genital femoral nerve and the ilioinguinal nerve. One must be aware that these structures are nearby, and always be cautious. I prevent injury to them by doing the dissection with loops, and when I visualize the cord, I know that the nerve is nearby. The genital branch of the genitofemoral nerve runs inside the cord and the ilioinguinal branch nerve is outside the cord.

I have never had a patient with any sensory loss of their penis, and I do not believe this technique leads to any erectile problems.

The angle of the erection, I believe, is overstated, and some people believe that when one divides the ligament, the angle of the erection becomes more obtuse. I have not found this to be the case.

Regarding other penile lengthening techniques, some state that you cannot cut all the ligament, as the angle of the erection will be affected. I believe this not to be correct. One can go ahead and divide all the ligament without having significant changes to the angle of the erection.

CAN YOU EXPLAIN TO US HOW DO YOU DO THE ASSESSMENT ON A PATIENT ASKING FOR THIS PROCEDURE? CAN YOU GIVE US SOME GUIDELINES FOR CONSTRUCTING AN ASSESSMENT CHART?

The assessment of these patients is pretty simple. They obviously need to have normal penile anatomy, which most men have. What I usually do is to try to make a measurement of the penis. This can be quite variable, depending on numerous factors such as whether the person is cold or frightened. This is mainly for one's records and to have a comparison postoperatively. A normal penis should be 8–10 cm in the flaccid state and 10–12 cm in the stretched state. I believe I can achieve an increase in length of between 2 and 4 cm. Prospective patients need to know that there may be no lengthening increase, although this is very rare. Another important thing is to assess the fat bulk over the lateral aspect of the mons pubis to give one some idea of the amount of fat in the area for the fat flaps. This is usually not a problem.

One also needs to assess the amount of fat that can be harvested for fat grafting. Any areas are suitable donor sites, but the usual ones are the central abdomen and hips. Very thin people pose a problem for fat grafting, as sometimes there is not enough fat for covering the entire penile girth. I like to inject a minimum of 25 mL of washed fat. If I can only get ~15 mL, then I only inject the fat over the dorsal surface.

Instead of using fat, one can inject hyaluronic acid (HA) in the same plane as the one used for fat grafting. This can be expensive and is usually used when patients come just for girth increase. The HA is a temporary filler and lasts in the penis for a variable amount of time. Men do not need to have a general anesthetic for this, and they will not need to go to the operating room for HA injections. When HA is used, I recommend using it in the penile shaft only. I do not inject the glans penis with fat or HA, as over the glans there is no plane to inject as there is over the penile shaft. The skin over the glans is firmly adherent to the deep fascia. I perform HA injections for the penile shaft in my office under a dorsal penile block.

There are no differences whether the penis is circumcised or not. I perform the same operation in both, although the fat grafting of the foreskin is a little bit more problematic. One needs to be quite conservative in putting a lot of fat into the foreskin. I found that because the skin is quite thin and there are two layers of this thin skin over this area that one can get some unevenness of the contour in the foreskin. One thus needs to be quite careful when putting fat into the foreskin. I also find that fat take seems to be less in the foreskin than around the shaft.

CAN YOU DESCRIBE YOUR TECHNIQUE?

My technique starts with the division of the suspension ligament.

I like to do the lengthening part first and this I do by designing a distally based V–Y advancement flap with the wide edges of the V being on each side of the proximal part of the dorsal penis shaft.

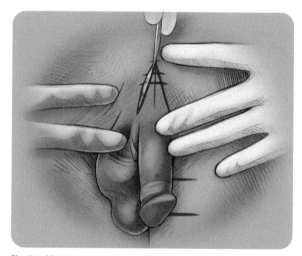

Fig. 8.1 Marking of the V–Y advancement flap.

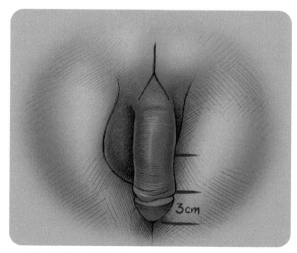

Fig. 8.2 Wound after closure of the V–Y advancement flap.

The sharp point of the V extends up to just short of where the hair finishes. I take care not to make the pointy end of the V–Y advancement flap too narrow for fear of distal flap necrosis. I then incise the flap down to the superficial fascia. I elevate the flap on the superficial fascia, and this preserves the blood supply of the V–Y advancement flap. I then extend the incision down to the deep fascia until I get onto the dorsal penile shaft. Occasionally, I come across the dorsal vein of the penis, which I usually like to preserve. This is not essential.

I then progress to divide the suspensory ligament as much as I can. I progress down the dorsal penile shaft until the symphysis pubis takes an upward turn. This dissection is rather deep. I use a lighted retractor to perform this dissection. As the pubis takes an upward turn, the dorsal penile nerves and veins are better visualized and become more apparent. The plane of dissection is relatively avascular. I have never used a drain in this area.

After I have divided the suspensory ligament, I progress to harvest the distally based inguinal/spermatic cord fat flaps. I take some of the superficial fat and then blend it around with the fat from around the spermatic cords. I need to get enough flap volume and mobility of this flap to be able to fill the depths of the dead space that has been created. I do this on each side of the penile shaft.

I then use a 2-0 PDS II (polydioxanone) suture to pick up some periosteum at the depth of the pubic symphysis to hold and direct the fat flaps into the base of the dead space. I then close the wound up in layers.

I then progress to harvest the fat grafting, usually from the mid-abdominal area through a separate incision to that of the V–Y advancement flap incision. I do this to avoid having extra serous fluid collecting in the previously operated dead space. One can also harvest the fat from the hips if necessary. I do not believe that fat from one area is superior to another. I usually take

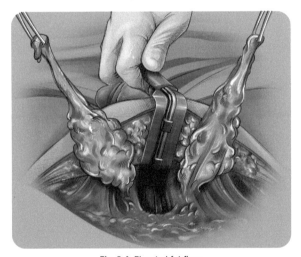

Fig. 8.4 Elevated fat flaps.

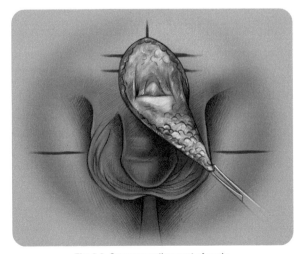

Fig. 8.3 Suspensory ligament of penis.

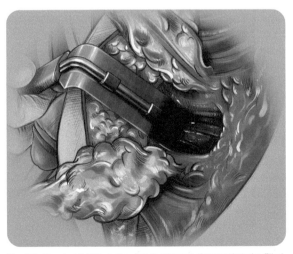

Fig. 8.5 Elevated fat flaps showing dead space that needs to be filled.

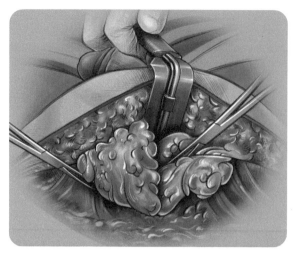

Fig. 8.6 Flaps tucked into dead space.

the fat from the mid lower abdominal area because people usually carry more fat there.

For the fat grafting, I harvest microfat. I use a cannula with fine holes. I wash the fat with saline over a sieve.

To inject the fat, I make a puncture hole with a 19 gauge sharp hypodermic needle over the dorsal penis shaft. I inject the fat through a single-hole 1.8 mm cannula and I place a few other holes over the proximal dorsal penile shaft and inject all the way down to the corona. I then make some small puncture incisions on the mid shaft to get fat into the proximal penile shaft and then do the same on the ventral surface. The fat is injected all the way around in two planes. The first pass is done on the tunica and then when this space is filled up, I direct my cannula in the subdermal plane. If the patient is too thin and I can only harvest about 15–17 mL of fat, then I inject all the fat on the dorsum. The minimum amount of fat to be injected is 25 mL of clean fat, but the more you inject, the better. I have injected up to 60–70 mL into the penis.

HOW CAN WE AVOID COMPLICATIONS?

Complications can be avoided, as in any operation, by knowing the anatomy and by being meticulous with the operating technique. Firstly, in the V–Y advancement flap, the flap must not be too thin, and one must elevate it to the level of the superficial fascia, that is, Scarpa's fascia.

The second aspect to take into account is when one elevates the V–Y advancement flap and as one dissects

over the dorsal penile shaft, one needs to know the anatomy in that area and stay away from the dorsal nerves of the penis and not injure them. If these are injured, the patient will have some numbness over the penis. If the more proximal nerve is damaged, this will result in erectile problems. There is a nice dissection plane over the penile dorsum. One needs to stay in this plane. When reaching the depth of the pubic bone, this is the closest that one will come to the dorsal penile nerves and veins. When the pubic bone turns upwards and the veins and nerves become visible, one needs to stop the dissection, as injury to the nerves and veins become too great.

The third thing is when elevating the fat flaps around the spermatic cord, I usually dissect with loops. One must differentiate between the pericord fat and the cord. One needs to be conscious of the change in anatomy from fat to spermatic cord to avoid damaging the cord structures.

Regarding the change in penis erection angle, there is no real problem with this in my experience. I always tell patients that this might occur.

Regarding the fat injections into the penis, the fat needs to be injected in the various layers and not just injected in a bolus. This is obviously beneficial for graft take. Harvesting microfat is better than harvesting big lobules of fat when it comes to skin smoothness. The skin is so thin over the penile shaft that you might see undulations and irregularities when not done properly.

Skin necrosis is not a problem with fat grafting. Necrosis of the fat flaps is very rare, since they are well vascularized.

After the procedure, the patient is covered with antibiotics. Infection is a low risk.

CAN YOU SUMMARIZE YOUR FOLLOW-UP AND PATIENT RECOMMENDATIONS?

This operation can be done as a day procedure. The procedure is done under general anesthesia and I use a dorsal penile block for postoperative analgesia. I find this useful for all penile surgery. Patients are discharged with analgesia.

With regard to the penis, I do not wrap the penis, but only dress the V–Y advancement flap wound. I leave this dressing intact for 10 days. I let the patients shower the next day and I cover the patients with oral antibiotics (cephalosporin) for 5 days.

I do not give the patients any antierection medication. If they have an erection, it can be painful, but they soon lose it. I tell them to refrain from any sexual activity for 3 weeks. This is mainly because of the fat grafting. I also ask patients not to exercise for 3 weeks. I apply a pressure garment for 2–3 weeks in the area where the fat was harvested.

There will be significant swelling of the penis that will remain for a couple of weeks. The penis will be firm for 6–8 weeks as a result of the fat grafting, but it will soften up after 2–3 months. I do not tell them to massage at all.

With regard to any follow-up fat grafting, this can be performed 4–6 months after the original operation. I do not believe that it is in anyone's interest to redo the suspensory ligament division unless they come from elsewhere and one is not sure of how much of the ligament has been divided.

Reabsorption of the fat is about 50%. Generally, I dislike making the girth of the penile shaft wider than the girth of the corona of glans penis. I feel that this does not look natural. I do not inject the glans penis to make it wider.

WHY DO YOU THINK THIS TECHNIQUE SHOULD BE IN THE ARMAMENTARIUM OF ANY PLASTIC SURGEON?

I think we plastic surgeons are better equipped to have this in our armamentarium because I believe we are more meticulous dissectors, and understand and dissect flaps better than urologists and general surgeons. This goes hand in hand with other plastic surgery procedures such as labiaplasties, which I believe are better performed by plastic surgeons than gynecologists because we give much more attention to detail. I also believe that these operations should be in our domain, although not many plastic surgeons do penile augmentation at the present time.

WHAT TIPS CAN YOU GIVE US TO INCLUDE THIS PROCEDURE IN OUR PRACTICE AND HOW TO MARKET IT?

I am not a marketing person. I do not market my practice. I believe if people are interested in this procedure, they will find it on our website, and they will make inquiries about it. Obviously, one can market this heavily and of course this can bring more people to your practice, but it might be detrimental to one's reputation.

This procedure can be a complement for body definition surgery in men but does not need to go hand in hand. Some people who want to look aesthetically better and svelte might not be worried about having a longer penis.

There are some insecurities that affect men, this being one of them. Most of the men who I see in consultation for penile augmentation have an average length penis. Their sexual function is good. Having a longer and thicker penis would make them feel better and more confident about themselves. They would feel more manly having a bigger penis.

Taking anabolic steroids decreases the size of a person's testicles but not the size of their penis. Their libido, however, is affected by taking these hormones. This operation does not improve the size of the testicles nor does it improve their libido.

Even within the transgender population, in the male-to-female transgender person, you can see when the transgender male has been on hormones for years; the size of the penis remains much the same.

Scrotal Reduction

An adjunctive procedure is that of a scrotal reduction.

This is a fairly simple operation. I like to make the incision in the midline raphe. One resects skin and dartos muscle. If one would like the scrotum to be elevated, the incision needs to be carried around the inferior aspect of the scrotum. One needs to

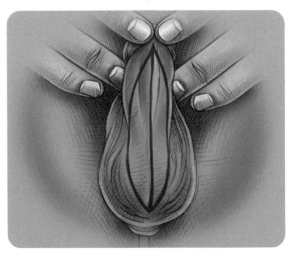

Fig. 8.7 Makings for scrotal reduction.

close the dartos muscle well as well as the skin. The resultant scar is good and mimics the midline scrotal raphe.

Penile Scrotal Webbing

I occasionally get asked by men if I can do something to improve how their scrotal skin extends onto their proximal penile shaft. An operation can improve this penile scrotal webbing. It can have the visual effect of having a longer penile shaft and generally making the penile scrotal area look better.

The operation is fairly simple, as with the procedure I perform for scrotal reduction. It leaves a well-hidden linear scar in the midline raphe.

The markings are basically an ellipse starting at the proximal point of the webbing. The amount of skin to be removed around the penis is assessed so as not to make the closure too tight.

I then continue the incision at a right angle over the scrotum, so the proximal and distal areas of the incisions are graded so as to minimize dog ears. The wound is closed in layers.

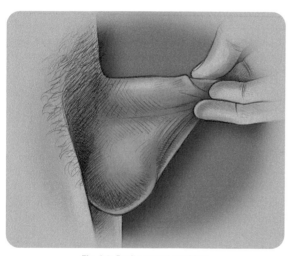

Fig. 8.8 Penile scrotal webbing.

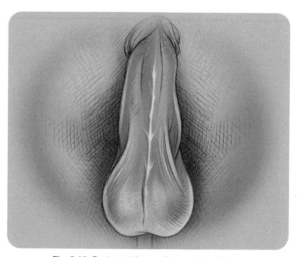

Fig. 8.10 Postoperative penile scrotal webbing.

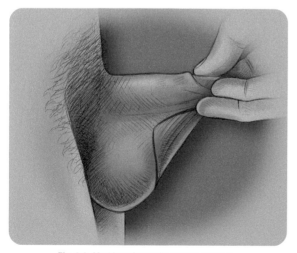

Fig. 8.9 Markings for penile scrotal webbing.

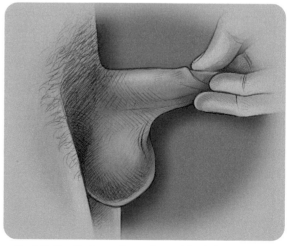

Fig. 8.11 Resultant scar after penile scrotal webbing correction.

Expert Profile

David Caminer
Plastic Surgeon
Sydney, Australia

David Caminer is a senior plastic and reconstructive surgeon affiliated with St. Vincent's Private and Public Hospital, Sydney, as well as East Sydney Private Hospital. He established the Head and Neck Reconstruction and Microsurgical unit at St. Vincent's Hospital, Sydney and specializes in a wide variety of plastic and reconstructive fields ranging from basic skin cancer removal and reconstruction to microsurgery, hand surgery, cosmetic surgery, genital surgery, and most recently in transgender surgery. He has always been involved in teaching students, residents, and registrars since the beginning his consultant career, and has been integral in teaching of fellows in the nuances of plastic surgery.

KEY ACHIEVEMENTS

Total Tracheal Reconstruction – "A World's First" November 1999.

Front Page, Sydney Morning Herald, Channel Seven News, Good Medicine.

Description of the CROWN flap. Used mainly for reconstruction of small defects of the extremities.

Description of a new technique for passing/tunneling the microvascular pedicle, popularizing the lateral arm free flap in head and neck reconstruction.

World's first tracheal reconstruction.

Description of the anatomy of the distal facial nerve.

Description of the new nipple reconstruction technique.

Description of reconstruction of bilateral maxillary defect with lateral arm osteocutaneous free flap.

Initiating the Plastic Surgery Fellowship program at St Vincent's Hospital, Sydney.

EDUCATION

2001 Medical Licensure: General License NSW Australia Renewal.

1995 Laser Course, Boston and Indianapolis, USA.

1993 FMGEMS 1 and 2, (American Medical Licensing Exam).

1993 FRACS (Plastic Surgery)–Australia.

1985 AMEC Medical Licensure: General License, NSW, Australia.

1982 MB, BCh., Bachelor of Medicine, Bachelor of Surgery, Medical.

School University of Witwatersrand, Johannesburg, South Africa.

1976 Matriculation, Marist Brothers College, Johannesburg, South Africa.

PROFESSIONAL EXPERIENCE

2014 – Present Head of Department of Plastic Surgery, East Sydney Private Hospital.

2000–2002 Secretary of NSW Chapter of Plastic and Reconstructive Surgery, St. Vincent's Hospital, Sydney.

1999–2006 Chairman and CSU Head, Department of Plastic and Reconstructive Surgery, St. Vincent's Hospital, Sydney.

1995–2006 VMO Plastic Surgeon, St. Vincent's Hospital, Sydney.

2006–Present HMO Plastic Surgeon, St. Vincent's Hospital, Sydney General Medical.

TRAINING

1983 Internship, general surgery.

General medicine, Obstetrics and Gynaecology, Baragwanath Hospital, Johannesburg, South Africa.

1984 Senior house officer, Plastic and Reconstructive Surgery, Johannesburg General Hospital and Hillbrow Hospital, Johannesburg, South Africa.

1984 Immigration to Australia.

1984 Surgical resident medical officer, General Surgery, Launceston General Hospital, Launceston, Tasmania, Australia.

Sydney Plastic Surgery Training Program.

1991 St. Vincent's Hospital, Plastic Surgery Unit.

1992 Concord Repatriation Hospital, Plastic Surgery Unit.

1993 Westmead Hospital, Plastic Surgery Unit.

Fellowships in Plastic Surgery

1994–1995 Cleveland Clinic Florida, Plastic Surgery Unit, Fort Lauderdale, Florida, USA.

Cleveland Clinic, Cleveland, Ohio, USA.

1995–1996 Professor J. Baudet/Professor Martin Bordeaux, France.

Employment as VMO

2010 – Present HMO Plastic and Reconstructive Surgery, St. Vincent's Public Hospital.

1995–2010 VMO Plastic and Reconstructive Surgery, St. Vincent's Public Hospital.

1999–2010 Growing the Reputation in Head and Neck Reconstruction, St. Vincent's Public Hospital.

1999–2006 Chairman of the Department of Plastic and Reconstructive Surgery, St. Vincent's Public Hospital.

1996–1999 Supervisor of plastic surgery training, St. Vincent's Public Hospital.

Research Projects

Conservative Management of Perforated Peptic Ulcers. Presented by Dr. Hogg at the Conference of Winter Medicine, St Anton, Austria, 1989.

Emergency Free Flaps at the Prince of Wales Hospital. Presented at the NSW Chapter of Plastic Surgeons, June 1990.

Selected for Poster Presentation, Registrars Paper Day, August 1990.

PUBLICATIONS

Barnouti L, Caminer D. Maxillary tumors and bilateral reconstruction of the maxilla, *ANZ J Surg.* 2006;76(4):267-269.

Caminer DM, Newman MI, Boyd JB. Angular nerve: new insights on innervation of the corrugator supercilii and procerus muscles, *J Plast Reconstr Aesthet Surg.* 2006;59:366-372.

Moisidis E, Caminer D. Osteocutaneous lateral arm flap reconstruction; a clinical review and laboratory study, *ANZ J Surg.* 2006;76(Suppl.):A60.

Shoshani OJ, Caminer D. The use of octyl-2-cyanoacrylate (Dermabond) in plastic surgery, *ANZ J Surg.* 2005;75(Suppl.):A90.

Merten S, Jiang RP, Caminer D. Submental artery island flap for head and neck reconstruction, *ANZ J Surg.* 2002;72:121-124.

Moon H, Caminer D, Boyd JB, Peroneal wounds. In: Wexner SD, Vernava AM, eds. *Clinical Decision Making in Colorectal Surgery.* Igaku-Shoin Publishers, 1995.

Boyd JB, Caminer D, PRS Book Review. In: Myers A, ed. *Biological Basis for Facial Plastic Surgery.* New York Thieme Medical; 1993.

PRESENTATIONS

Endoscopic brow lifting – Presented at NSW Chapter meeting 2016.

Clinical and Pathological Characteristics of Incompletely Excised Basal Cell Carcinomas, 32nd Annual Meeting of Israeli Society of Plastic Surgeons. November 2005, Israel.

Maxillary Tumours and Bilateral Reconstruction of the Maxilla, Dr. Laith Barnuti, Dr. David Caminer. Presented at IPRAS, Sydney, 2003.

The Crown Flap – A New Radial Random Pattern Flap, Maroshnik M, Caminer D, Australian ASC, 2003.

Hand Function Following Radial Artery Harvesting, AC Thompson, P Spratt, D Caminer, Departments of Cardiothoracic and Plastic Surgery, St. Vincent's Hospital, Sydney. Presented at the Affiliate Symposium of the Annual Scientific Meeting of the Cardiac Society of Australia and New Zealand, Melbourne, August 2000.

A New Nipple Reconstruction – The "Kiss" Principle. Canadian Society Plastic and Reconstructive Surgery Meeting, Saskatchewan, Canada 1995, Australian Society of Aesthetic Plastic Surgery, Port Douglas, 1999.

Suction Assisted Passage of a Microsurgical Pedicle, AGM Australasian College of Surgeons, Sydney, 1999.

Maxillary Reconstruction Using Calvarial Bone Graft and Myofascial Rectus Abdominus Free Flap, AGM Australasian College of Surgeons, Sydney, 1999.

The Facial Nerve Beyond the Parotid, American Society of Plastic and Reconstructive Surgery, San Francisco, California, USA, 1997.

Augmentation Phalloplasty – ISAPS Conference, Brisbane, Australia, October 2019.

Pearls in Abdominoplasty – ASAPS Conference, Brisbane, Australia, October, 2019.

BIBLIOGRAPHY

Alter GJ: Augmentation phalloplasty, *Urol Clin North Am.* 22: 887–902, 1995.

da Ros C, Teloken C, et al. Caucasian penis: what is normal size? Presented at the American Urological Association 89th Annual Meeting, San Francisco, May 16, 1994.

Kelley JH, Eraklis AJ: A procedure for lengthening the phallus in boys with exstrophy of the bladder, *J Pediatric Surg.* 6:645–649, 1971.

Kim JJ, Kwak TI, Jeon BG, Cheon J, Moon DG: Human glans penis augmentation using injectable hyaluronic acid gel, *Int J Impot Res.* 15(6):439–443, 2003.

Long DC: Elongation of the penis. [In Chinese.], *Chung Hua Cheng Hsing Shoa Shang Wai Ko Tsa Chih* 6:17–19, 1990.

Nguyen PS, Desouches C, Gay AM, Hautier A, Magalon G: Development of micro-injection as an innovative autologous fat graft technique: the use of adipose tissue as dermal filler, *J Plast Reconstr Aesthet Surg.* 65:1692–1699, 2012.

Reich J: The aesthetic surgical experience. In Smith JW, Aston SJ, editors: *Smith and Grabb's Plastic Surgery*, 4th ed., Boston, 1991, Little, Brown and Company, pp 127.

Roos H, Lissoos I: Penis lengthening, *Int J Aesthetic Restorative Surg* 2:89–96, 1994.

Trepsat F: Midface reshaping with micro-fat grafting. [In French.], *Ann Chir Plast Esthet.* 54:435–443, 2009.

Chapter 9

Fat Grafting to the Penis

Dr. Theodore Vodoukis

Plastic Surgeon, Greece

Chapter Outline

Why Did You Decide to Do This Technique?

When Did You Learn It? Historically, What Is Your Contribution?

Can This Technique Be Compared To Others and Why?

Expert Approach: Fat Grafting to the Penis

How did you end up doing it?

Can this technique be compared to others and why?

What do you consider to be important landmarks and anatomy to be able to better perform this technique?

Can you explain to us how you do the assessment on a patient asking for this procedure?

Can you describe your technique?

Can you share with us any complications?

Can you summarize your follow-up?

Why do you think this technique should be in the armamentarium of any plastic surgeon?

What tips can you give us to include this procedure in our practice?

Expert Profile

Why Did You Decide to Do This Technique?

Penis enlargement is becoming more popular every day and thousands of male individuals are seeking some help to satisfy their desire.

Our community, however, is generally skeptical of performing penile enlargements because of the uncertain results and bad reputation, mostly produced by non-board-certified plastic surgeon physicians or unprepared medical professionals and commercial agencies, who reproduce and imitate the penis enlargement surgical procedure. Many individuals have ended up dissatisfied, with severe complications, because they have been offered paramedical, practical, surgical, or nonsurgical therapies and have been cheated with treatment options without a doubt are not in the armamentarium of any ethical plastic surgeon or even respectful physician.

We never put any pressure on an individual to proceed with this operation. It is his sovereign decision whether to proceed or not. We should never promise results that surpass the capability of our technique. Patients with unrealistic expectations, who request results superior to those explained, or who feel entitled to obtain the maximum penile increase based on ideas and perceptions coming from adult videos, should be excluded.

But before we start analyzing the plastic surgery methods that enhance penis enlargement, we need to review the physiological function and size of the penis, the history, anatomy, and histology for this operation.

When Did You Learn It? Historically, What Is Your Contribution?

In 1982, a French plastic surgeon, Yve Gerard Ylouz, was probably the first to *liporecycle* fat microparticles (lipoaspirates), for cosmetic purposes. That was performed on a young actress, a close friend of Ylouz, by aspirating the fat cells of a lipoma on her back, using a very small liposuction cannula and transferring the lipoaspirate as it was, to the deep nasolabial folds. I was present as an assistant young plastic surgeon at this historical procedure and at many more to follow, evaluating and developing the lipotransfer technique. We used the term liporecycling, interpreted from the Greek *Λίπο ανακύκλωση* (*leapo anakeek-clossi*), meaning literally recycling the fat. In 1983, at the BAAPS course in London, together with Bryan Mayou, we presented officially (*ISAPS Newsletter,* September–December 2012, 27–29), maybe the first in the UK, the new technique of liposuction and a few years later, lipotransfer of lipoaspirates. After that year, liporecycling became maybe the most wanted, frequent, and popular plastic surgery procedure and ever since, plastic surgeons all over the world have reliably used fat grafting as a way to improve and enhance cosmetic appearance or augment many anatomical areas. Either as a core procedure or an adjunct to several other plastic reconstructive or cosmetic surgery procedures on breast, face, scalp, feet, hands, hips, buttocks, and endless other anatomical sites, today liporecycling remains within the top five plastic surgery procedures.

Two major disappointment in those early years was that the transplanted fat was short surviving and that the fat could not be preserved for later second-time use. Over the last 15–20 years, plastic surgeons started, and then clinicians followed, to document in several publications the therapeutic benefits of fat grafting with or without added platelet-rich plasma (PRP) and adipose tissue-derived stem cells (ATSCs, which are present of course in the stromal vascular fraction, [SVF]).

Given today's answers and knowledge, during that time of the late '70s and early '80s, fat recycling was the subject of extended studies and strong discussions, and considered the hot topic for congresses and scientific panels. As well, at the same time, as plastic surgeons, we received vast amounts of ironic comments and dispute, unfortunately not only from other physicians, but sadly from conservative or skeptical members of our own society.

Nowadays, many other non-plastic surgery specialties are using liporecycling to assist their procedures and enhance their therapeutic results. Gynecology, orthopedics, urology, ophthalmic surgery, ENT, dermatology, and of course, general surgery are among those specialties using fat in addition to the most commonly done plastic surgeries.

In fat-grafting history, we see the names of Gustav Neuber (1850–1932 German plastic surgeon) and Dr. Viktor Czerny, a German Bohemian surgeon, who at the beginning of the early 20th century used lipografting not as harvested fat micro lipoaspirates, but as an entire lipoma or a fat-piece transfer. In fact, fat grafting at the beginning indeed had trouble gaining acceptance, mainly for its poor results, as modern liposuction techniques had not yet been developed or standardized, and there was a lack of experience and knowledge.

Fat grafting should be performed in a hospital or outpatient surgery center, and when done in private consultation facilities, only as where they are accredited. Facility accreditation is important as it guarantees that the specific facility is inspected at regular intervals by the public health authorities or ministry, ensuring patient safety, best practices, and that operations are performed by certified plastic surgeons.

Can This Technique Be Compared To Others and Why?

Surgical penis enlargement and elongation methods include various types of penile augmentation and suspensory ligament release. Penile augmentation involves injecting mostly fat cells or other types of injectables into the penis, or grafting dermofat pieces. Injecting fat cells into the penis is the most common technique.

When done by inexperienced physicians, fat transfer, fillers injection, and placing dermo-fat grafts into the penis (usually to the dorsum) can cause severe deformity and functional issues, which, in some instances, are long-lasting or unrepairable. Suspensory ligament surgery produces a high rate of functional issues. All those surgeries leave scarring at the operation and donor site and the results in size may disappear over a short time, leaving calcified tissue. For the recipient individual, this is a most uncomfortable and unpleasant situation that demands extrusion and correction, which sometimes is not very successful.

Suspensory ligament release increases flaccid penis length, but does not increase by any means the length of an erect penis and usually because of the instability that this operation produces, creates firmness problems with sexual dysfunction. The suspensory ligament is the remainder in mankind of the erectile bone in canids (dogs, wolves, and many more carnivores, household or wild). Functionally, the suspensory ligament supports and maintains the base of the penis attached to the pubis. It is the main point of support and straightening for the erect penis, keeping it in an upright and stable position during sexual intercourse.

Expert Approach: Fat Grafting to the Penis

Theodore Vodoukis
Plastic Surgeon
Athens, Greece

HOW DID YOU END UP DOING IT?

We must emphasize that the initiative of this study was to assist plastic surgeons when counseling patients considering or asking for penile cosmetic surgery (for length and circumference augmentation) and to provide them with guidelines on the technique to perform the best possible operation and obtain optimum results.

CAN THIS TECHNIQUE BE COMPARED TO OTHERS AND WHY?

There are several surgical or nonsurgical penis enlargement treatments, most of which carry a risk of significant complications and give no results, especially when performed by unlicensed physicians, which can lead to disaster.

The American Urological Association (AUA) and the Urology Care Foundation "consider subcutaneous fat injection for increasing penile girth to be a procedure which has not been shown to be safe or efficacious. The AUA also considers the division of the suspensory ligament of the penis for increasing penile length in adults to be a procedure which has not been shown to be safe or efficacious." Also, complications from penis enlargement procedures using dermo-fat,

are the worst, including scarring that may lead, eventually, to penis shrinkage or erectile dysfunction.

Other surgical treatments include the injection of dermal fillers, silicone gel, or poly(methyl methacrylate)—PMMA. All those methods are also not approved, not only by the US Food and Drug Administration (FDA) for use in the penis, but also are mostly refused by serious professionals.

A 2019 study in *Sexual Medicine Reviews* found that nonsurgical methods of penis enlargement are typically ineffective and can be damaging to both physical and mental health. The authors found that such treatments are "supported by scant, low-quality evidence, unethical advertisement, fake statistics, news and rumors."

Injectable pharmacological drugs (papaverine) and fat transfer surgery should remain the best options, considered as the only ethical procedures, and all others should remain in clinical trials.

Again, according to the 2019 study in Sexual Medical Reviews, Overall, other treatments' outcomes performed by non-specialized physicians, were from little acceptance to poor, with low satisfaction rates and significant risk of major complications, including penile deformity, shortening, and erectile dysfunction."

Without commenting on those reviews, even if they are coming from the most reputable entities, we will concentrate on the plastic surgery options, as plastic surgery is the core knowledge in the area of penis enlargement. Offering the most advanced combined techniques of fat transfer, that really have changed the results and statistics, posturing acceptable long-lasting results, cover the up to now lack of a reliable method for this operation.

Fat transfer or liporecycling for penis enlargement (also referred to as fat grafting or fat injections), is the surgical process by which fat is harvested and implanted from one area of the body to the penis of the same individual. The objective is to augment, correct, or support the area where the fat is injected. The technique involves extracting adipose fat by means of mini-liposuction, processing the fat in-house (international regulations prohibit the transport of collected fat outside of the surgery premises for further processing), and then reinjecting it into the penis. We have concluded that injecting fat together with PRP, fat tissue stem cells (FTSCs), which exist mostly in the SVF, all prepared at the same time in the operating theater, gives much better and longer-lasting results, contradicting the theory of a nonviable operation.

WHAT DO YOU CONSIDER TO BE IMPORTANT LANDMARKS AND ANATOMY TO BE ABLE TO BETTER PERFORM THIS TECHNIQUE?

Histology

Fat tissue consists of three main types of fat or adipose cells. An average human adult has 30 billion fat cells with a weight of 30 pounds, or 13.5 kg. If excess weight is gained as an adult, fat cells increase in size about fourfold before dividing and increasing the absolute number of fat cells present. Of major importance is the fact that the proportion of volume to weight of fat is not 1:1. One cubic centimeter of fat weighs 0.7–0.8 g.

White Fat Cells (Unilocular Cells). A typical fat cell is 0.1 mm in diameter, with some being twice that size and others half that size. White fat cells contain a large lipid droplet surrounded by a layer of cytoplasm. The nucleus is flattened and located on the periphery. The fat stored is in a semiliquid state and is composed primarily of triglycerides and cholesteryl ester. White fat cells secrete many proteins acting as adipokines, such as resistin, adiponectin, leptin, and apelin.

Brown Fat Cells (Multilocular Cells). These are polyhedral in shape. Unlike white fat cells, these cells have considerable cytoplasm, with lipid droplets scattered throughout. The nucleus is round, and, although eccentrically located, it is not in the periphery of the cell. The brown color comes from a large number of mitochondria. Brown fat, also known as "baby fat," is used to generate energy in several forms.

Marrow Fat Cells (Unilocular Cells). Marrow adipocytes, like brown and white adipocytes, are derived from mesenchymal stem cells.

The marrow adipose tissue deposit is poorly understood in terms of its physiologic function and relevance to bone health. Marrow adipose tissue expands in situations of low bone density, but additionally, it expands in the setting of obesity.

Since the new millennium, several groups of plastic surgeons and researchers from all over the world have already published many papers on tissue engineering, describing the implications and assistance of adipose tissue in the new cell-based regenerative therapies. This was quite a revelation and at the same time a relief to the scientific community, as up until the last century, adult mesenchymal stem cells (MSCs) were thought to exist predominantly as a bone marrow product. As it turns out in the last decades, adipose tissue is a much more rich, perpetual, and prolific source of MSCs than bone marrow. By volume, MSCs are actually 300–500 times more plentiful in adipose tissue as compared with bone marrow tissue. Together with the ease of harvesting and extraction of adipose tissue (compared with bone marrow), this opened up a whole new chapter in the field of reconstructive and regenerative plastic surgery.

A Normal or Acceptable Size for the Penis

Although results vary slightly across reputable studies, the accepted mean for the human penis, when erect, varies within the range of 12.9–15 cm (5.1–5.9 in) in length. It is not necessarily correlated with anthropometric measurements such as height, weight, and body mass index (BMI).

In a systematic review published in the *International British Journal of Urology* by Veale et al. (2015), covering the previous 30 years research on the topic, they presented data showing almost similar results, giving mean penis lengths when flaccid of 9.16 cm, stretched nonerect of 13.24 cm, and erect of 13.12 cm respectively, and mean flaccid or erect circumferences (girth) of 9.31 cm and 11.66 cm respectively.

The most important factor that affects penile dimensions, beyond any doubt or skepticism, is the arousal and the frequency of arousal during every man's whole life. Sexual arousal, also called sexual excitement or desire, is typically and literally what men want during or in anticipation and expectancy of sexual activity. A number of physiological reactions occur mainly in the mind and consecutively to the body as preparation for sexual intercourse and continue during it. Male arousal will lead under any circumstances to an erection; that is a simple biological pattern. The female arousal response involves sexual tissues such as nipples, vulva, clitoris, vaginal walls, and vaginal lubrication, having a more complicated pattern. Mental and physical stimuli such as touch, odor, view, and the internal fluctuation of hormones influence and maintain sexual arousal. Sexual arousal has several stages and may not lead always to any actual sexual activity, apart from mental arousal and the physiological changes that come with it. Given sufficient sexual stimulation, sexual arousal in humans reaches its climax during an orgasm. It may also be pursued for its own sake, even in the absence of an orgasm, especially for youngsters.

However, the relationship between erection and arousal is not one-to-one. After their mid-fifties (depending as well on the culture of the individual), men report that they do not always have an erection when they are sexually aroused or challenged.

Length When Flaccid. The length of the flaccid penis does not necessarily mirror the length of the erect penis; some smaller flaccid penises become much longer, whereas some larger flaccid penises show comparatively less elongation.

Owing to the action of the complex cremaster muscle-ligament, the penis and scrotum can contract involuntarily in response to cold temperatures, fear, nervousness, and anxiety, referred to by the slang term "shrinkage." The same phenomenon affects men who sit all day during their jobs, drivers, cyclists, and exercise bike users who receive prolonged pressure on the perineum from the chair, driving seat, bicycle, or saddle. The lack of exercise, movement, or standing causes the penis and scrotum to contract involuntarily. An incorrect seat or long sitting in a saddle may eventually cause erectile dysfunction.

Length When Stretched. In 2015, a study of 15,521 men found that the average length of a stretched flaccid penis was 13.24 cm (5.21 inches) long. This is nearly indistinguishable from the average length of an erect human penis, which is 13.12 cm (5.17 inches) long, meaning that more or less, a stretched flaccid penis only changes in girth when erect.

Neither age, ethnicity, or size of the flaccid penis could accurately foresee erectile length. But stretched (when flaccid) length has a notable correlation with erect length, although we have not seen drastic differences between stretched and erect lengths.

An Italian study of around 3300 men published in *European Urology* concluded that flaccid stretched length on average measured about 12.5 cm (4.9 in), while an erect human penis is 13.12 cm (5.17 inches) long. In addition, when they checked for correlations in a random group of the same sample consisting of 325 men, they found statistically a very slight linear correlation (Spearman). Significant correlations exist between flaccid length and height of -0.208, weight -0.140, and -0.238 with BMI (flaccid circumference and height of -0.156, -stretched length and height -0.221, weight -0.136, BMI -0.169). As Spearman's correlation is NOT a linear one, we do not expect that a man with a high BMI to always have a relatively bigger and wider penis.

In statistics, Spearman's rank correlation coefficient, denoted by the Greek letter ρ (rho), is a nonparametric measure of rank correlation (statistical dependence between the rankings of two variables).

When Erect. Studies relying on self-measurement, including those from Internet surveys, consistently reported a higher average length than those using medical or scientific methods to obtain measurements. This emphasizes and provides evidence here of the personal psychological factor, self-esteem, and individual's point of view.

In a study of 80 healthy males, the average erect penis length was measured as 12.9 cm (5.1 in) (*Journal of Urology*, September 1996). Erection was pharmacologically induced in 80 physically normal American men (varying ethnicity, average age 54). It was concluded: "Neither patient age nor size of the flaccid penis can accurately predict erectile length."

A review published in the 2007 issue of *BJU International* showed the average erect penis length to be 14–16 cm (5.5–6.3 in) and girth to be 12–13 cm (4.7–5.1 in). The paper compared the results of 12 studies conducted on different populations in several countries.

An Indian study of 500 men aged 18–60 published in the *International Journal of Impotence Research* found, respectively, length to be: flaccid, 8.21 cm (3.23 in); stretched, 10.88 cm (4.28 in); and erect, 13.01 cm (5.12 in).

The most recent Korean study (published in 2016) of 248 Korean men identified the average erect penile length to be 13.53 cm (5.33 in).

All these citations are mentioned here to emphasize the fact of similarity in the penis dimensions, regardless of country, race, or other anthropomorphic values.

CAN YOU EXPLAIN TO US HOW YOU DO THE ASSESSMENT ON A PATIENT ASKING FOR THIS PROCEDURE?

It is not ethical or scientifically advisable, even against the physician's reputation, to proceed with penis enlargement to individuals suffering from diabetes, immunology and collagen diseases, coagulopathies, cardiopathies, neoplasia, individuals under chemoradiotherapy, infections in progress, those who had prior pelvic surgeries for urogenital conditions or trauma, severe systemic conditions, significant anxiety, distorted or not accepting of their sex (gender dysphoria needs entirely another plastic surgery approach), not accepting of their body image, with history of suicidal thoughts and/or attempted suicide linked to presumed genital inadequacy with psychogenic sexual dysfunction and psychiatric conditions under treatment.

Cases as well of true hypoplasia (micropenis), defined as a length of <2.5 cm relaxed, should follow another pathway of surveys and possible treatment.

It is an absolute contraindication to fat transfer patients taking immunosuppressive medications.

There are two types of individuals presenting in our offices seeking a procedure to have their penis surgically augmented:

(A) Those who are having really objective problems in size and girth based on reasonable reasons such as congenital, trauma, postsurgical complications, and time- and age-related conditions at the inconvenient moment (temperature, nervousness, and anxiety or psychological status).

(B) Men who have a normal-sized penis or even bigger, but who may experience penile dysmorphophobia by underestimating their own penis size while overestimating others' average penis size. Such dysmorphophobia is enhanced these days by the widely available circulation of pornographic movies mainly on the Web, showing extra-gifted individuals participating in those kinds of videos, but usually having pharmaceutically or technically induced big erect genitalia, rather than being a gifted man.

Both of those categories involve individuals who already have visited nonmedical professionals, asking for, or even having already had, surgical procedures, technical aids, or pharmacological treatments without, of course, getting any results. All those are mostly guided by fake scam advertisements.

CAN YOU DESCRIBE YOUR TECHNIQUE?
Penis Enlargement by Fat Grafting Process

It is strongly advisable that the individual's medical history be fully gathered and medical examination and tests are done (routine blood tests, X-ray, cardio), including an objective examination of the external genitalia, photos, and measurement of the length and circumference of the penis at rest (flaccid) and stretched. It is advisable to do a basal penile ultrasound scan to verify the presence of nodules, plaques, or lesions in the internal tissues of the penis.

PRP Preparation

Centrifugation: The Earth's gravitational force is sufficient to separate many types of particles if a substance remains motionless for several minutes. A tube of an anticoagulated blood sample left standing still on a benchtop will eventually separate into red blood cell (RBC) and white blood cell (WBC) fractions and plasma. However, the time required excludes this method of separation for most applications in the operating theater. In addition, the actual degradation of biological compounds during prolonged storage demands faster segmentation and separation techniques. Thus, to quicken sedimentation, the effect of gravity is amplified using centrifugal force, which can represent many thousand times the force of gravity.

We prefer to use the centrifuge PRP preparation method, as it is more economical, reliable, and quick.

We obtain a blood sample by venipuncture in acid citrate dextrose (ACD) tubes, a total of 30–40 mL.

Do not chill the blood at any time before or during platelet separation.

Centrifuge the blood using a "soft spin"; 300 rev/min for 6 minutes.

Three layers are separated because of different densities: the bottom layer consisting of RBCs, the middle layer consisting of platelets and WBCs, and the top the platelet-poor plasma (PPP) layer. The PPP layer should be collected and aseptically stored to be used to dilute the SVF later.

Transfer the middle section plasma, as it is the part that contains some platelets, into another sterile tube (without anticoagulant).

Centrifuge the tube at a higher speed (a hard spin) of 600 rev/min for at least 12 minutes to obtain a platelet concentrate.

The lower two thirds is the PRP and the upper third is again the remaining PPP that should be removed and stored with the first one. At the bottom of the tube, a dense pellet is formed.

Remove the PRP and carefully mix the remaining pellet with the preserved and stored aside PPP quantity of plasma (4–8 mL) by gently shaking the tube.

The layer of PRP prepared by centrifugation will be injected equally subcutaneously to the whole shaft surface, acting as a tissue separator (in between the skin and loose circumferential tissue and superficial and deep fascia layers), but mostly acting as a nutrient for the injected fat graft. The PPP will be used to dilute the SVF.

SVF (ATSCs) Preparation

It is emphasized that the preparation of all the endogenic factors should be done within the operating area where the fat and blood is collected. This is because of the international guidance and rules that apply to most countries: If any of the harvested fat or blood leaves the accredited operation theater area to be manipulated or processed elsewhere, it should be considered furthermore not as a surgical homogenous tool to complete the operation, but will enter the regulations as a prepared medication, subject to all pharmacological rules and approval.

Here there is a controversy. Surgical standards based upon a single operation on a single patient in an accredited operation theater differ significantly and by all means are higher than those from the Good Manufacturing Practices (GMP) standards, enforced in commercial pharmaceutical laboratories or companies for mass-produced pharmaceuticals. However, any manufactured drug is required at the end of the production line to be identical in constituents, purity, dose, strength, and be in mass production, whereas autologous SVF could never be produced and characterized that way. Every "amount" of produced SVF is individual, like its individual donor. The guarantee

for higher standards of the in-theater–produced SVF than those of an drug manufactured under GMP is also a matter of an accordingly equipped laboratory. Within the sterile area of the operating theater and, of course, with the aid of well-trained personnel (biologists, biochemists, or paramedics) who are qualified to produce on-site (with the necessary equipment) the absolutely essential materials for the transfer—PRP, SVF, ADSCs—the absolute highest quality of the product is indisputable. And, of course, this automatically comes under the domain of the plastic surgeon to produce and deploy the cells for their patient's benefit for a successful penis fat transfer.

In the vast majority of medical works, it is noted that the adipose tissue, or fat, is the source of SVF, but the truth is that it is not the adipose tissue, only the stromal part of the fat obtained in lipoaspirates (Greek στρώμα, "stroma," which means the layer, thereafter here the layers of loose connective tissue). Histologically, the fat lobules are encircled by loose connective tissue (stromal) and the SVF cells are present only in the loose connective tissue, which is also the home of capillaries and small vessels and not the fat tissue. Stromal tissue is a widely used histological term referring to loose connective tissue.

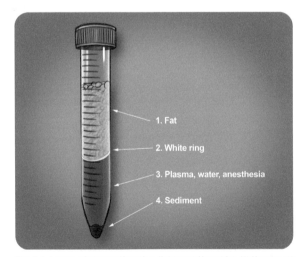

Fig. 9.1 Layers after centrifugation, light centrifuged fat: (1) Upper part oil/fat. (2) White ring (the little white ring at the bottom part of the fat is stroma produced only by the centrifugation, containing mostly collagen). (3) Watery part (local anesthetic and plasma). (4) At the very bottom, white and red blood cells and a small quantity of stromal vascular fraction.

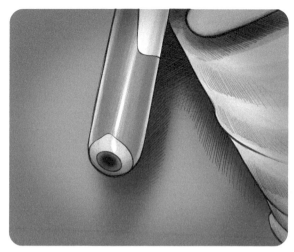

Fig. 9.2 Digested and centrifuged fat. The stromal vascular fraction is at the bottom.

Although there are a variety of methods for obtaining adipose SVF and the derived stem cells, the preferred author's method is using liposuction and segmentation by mixing collagenase 1A enzyme. It is an efficient and easy method that separates SVF only from the collagen stroma and also releases cells, providing the best variety and quality of stem cells.

Cytometric immunophenotyping tests in samples of autologous SVF demonstrate four distinctive intense stem cell lines, in varying percentage ratios, that include:

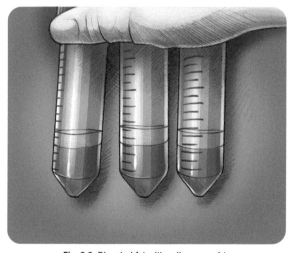

Fig. 9.3 Digested fat with collagenase A1.

(a) pericyte (lying around blood vessels) progenitor cells, (b) hematopoietic stem cells, (c) MSCs, and (d) endothelial progenitor cells. Autologous SVF also contains, in small amounts, non-progenitor cells such as T-reg cells, macrophages and epithelial cells. And of course in the more prominent layers of the autologous SVF we can see RBC's and WBC's and at the bottom we can also find the important mixture of cytokines. Similar findings have been reported in initial studies of SVF composition. SVF is organized by different cells, including a large amount of mesenchymal ATSCs, fibroblasts, endothelial cells, erythrocytes, vascular smooth muscle cells, hematopoietic cells, and other immune cells. The ATSCs can undergo multilineage differentiation and may be crucial for fat graft take, as it is common knowledge that mature adipocytes, even when surviving harvesting procedures, will not duplicate and take away the sooner or later and leave: will die within a few months, generating additionally harmful inflammatory responses and eventually causing the formation of connective tissue. Indeed, lipotransfer, when enriched with ATSCs insert (included in SVF), has been associated with better graft viability and surgical cosmetic outcome for a longer time.

Fat Harvesting—the Process Starts With Harvesting and Processing

Fat harvesting is performed from where the individual has more fat deposits, taking into consideration that the pubis, lower abdomen, and flank are the best sites in men and usually exist as secondary sex characteristics.

We use manual lipoaspiration by means of a 50 cc syringe, a stopper, and a lipocannula with multi-import holes, 2 or 3 mm width, 20 cm long, disposable or multiuse.

Attention should be taken to match the cannula import holes and syringe "neck" in diameter. The distal entrance holes should be smaller than the syringe entrance, hence allowing the fat cells to pass from the cannula to the syringe lumen freely, easily, comfortably, atraumatically, and without needing to apply a large force to obtain the negative pressure required. The syringe is better if it is the type that has an incorporated Luer lock screw, and the applied negative pressure must be enough to aspirate, but not damage and break the fat cells. The plunger should be retracted

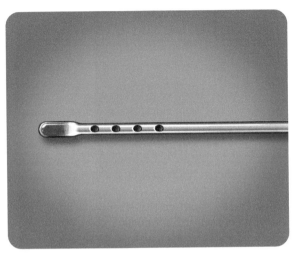

Fig. 9.4 Lipoaspiration cannula, 2mm width and 25cm long, with multiple holes.

to create a stabilized negative pressure within the syringe; then the retracted plunger should be locked so the subpressure remains well stabilized during the harvesting. We prefer as a traction locker, the type that has a syringe-inserted bar, with a metal mustache spring to lock in the upper distal edges of the syringe.

Part of the collected fat (up to 50 cc) will be processed as a source to obtain SVF and the rest of the fat (max 60 cc) as the initial volumizer. In the meantime, 25–30 cc of blood are collected and the procedure of the PRP preparation is started.

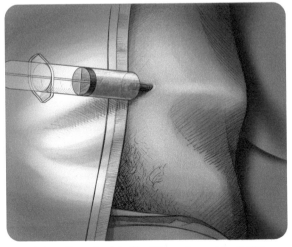

Fig. 9.5 Harvesting fat with a 50 cc syringe using a locker.

The whole procedure is performed under local anesthesia: lidocaine, ropivacaine for the penis, plus adrenaline 0.5 mg, for the harvesting site.

Lidocaine 2%, 50 mL, ropivacaine 7%, 10 mL (total solution 60 mL), 5 mL of the aforementioned solution without adrenaline, is used in its pure form to anesthetize the penis, while the rest is diluted in 250 mL of 0.9% sodium chloride with 0.5 mg of adrenaline and 10 mL of sodium bicarbonate for infiltration subcutaneously in the region where adipocytes will be harvested. We have used this solution since 1982.

We prefer the "regional block" local anesthesia to anesthetize the whole penis, by means of a "ring" pattern injection, in the base of the shaft, at the borders with the pubis, using deep infiltration in the whole zone as well as to the zone of the suspensory ligament of the penis. That anesthesia works for the whole penis surface within a maximum of 5 minutes and lasts for more than 6 hours. This technique avoids the injection of local anesthesia to the subcutaneous penile shaft where the fat graft will be placed, thus avoiding the excess edema and anatomical deterioration.

We implement light centrifugation or gravity separation of the fat meant to be used as a volumizer from the watery and oily part of the lipoaspirates. The watery part also contains local anesthesia from the donor site (a minimal amount of adrenaline), which nevertheless eventually produces vasoconstriction at the recipient's site, resulting in a severe delay to the initial and most important graft intake sequence. The intake and adaptation of the freshly transferred cells starts within the first 48 hours. In the meantime, the transferred fat cells are surviving from nutrients of the surrounding small quantities of plasma, having the PRP that was injected just before acting as a nutrient.

In our experience, this practice is much better, allowing standard surgical manipulations, lacking complications and major side effects, with less discomfort and morbidity. It is widely liked by patients and ensures brief, protected, and uneventful discharge time (120 ± 30 minutes) as an outpatient, including the administration procedure.

As a common practice, we always administer IV antibiotics (preferably second-generation cephalosporins) and sedation for the best comfort of these already anxious, worrying individuals. This sedation is not standardized, depending on the psychological status and of course, individual body weight. The maximum we usually administer is premedication midazolam 0.04–0.05 mg/kg.

During local anesthesia sedation with fentanyl 0.7–0.8 g/kg + propofol 0.8–1.6 mg/kg is used.

We always support the procedure with 250 mg of hydrocortisone stat at the beginning.

After the fat is collected, a maximum volume of 80–120 cc, it is separated into two sterile containers, the first containing 50 cc (maximum), which will serve for the important production of SVF. The rest (50–70 cc) will be processed with decanting or centrifugation (an alternate method is to wash the fat with a sterile saline solution) to separate debris, excess fluid, and dead cells from the viable adipose fat cells to be used immediately after as the volumizing matrix for the SVF acceptance–receiving region.

Fat is a delicate tissue and must be handled with maximal care to maintain its viability. Patient-related health conditions and factors should be taken into consideration when designing an operation for penis enlargement. The ideal methodology to approach autologous fat grafting has been, in the last years, a matter of constant discussion, where today we are still missing a common standard way to do it.

We have a principle in all of our work: The best technique is the one that any and each of us knows better and feels more secure to proceed with.

Even with all those years and between all the authors and studies, still there is no unanimously accepted harvesting technique that offers the highest and best quality collected fat while having less morbidity and fewer complications.

Nevertheless, let us review some interesting conclusions.

Distinct and different harvesting procedures result in different outcomes of fat graft take. As observed by multiple studies, in vitro and in vivo animal experiments, and further analysis, including human statistics, several variables need to be taken into account in order to come to a conclusion regarding the highest possible cell viability and survival rates.

The best sites from which to harvest and collect the fat are the places where the body accumulates more superficial adipose tissue (fat cells). Since the beginning of liporecycling history, it has been well known that lipoaspirate samples of either fat cells or

MSCs revealed a higher concentration of cells when collected from the lower abdomen (pubic area), inner thigh, and knee when compared with those collected from the upper abdomen, trochanteric region, and flank.

From our experience, we still support the idea that the richest and more efficient lipoaspirate is collected when harvesting lipomas, regardless of the site.

The absence of standardization in the protocols and the unpredictability of the survival of grafted tissues set a significant limitation for a commonly accepted technique to support the maximum possible graft retention and therefore the subsequent filling. Additionally, the lack of a standard assay to determine viability or volume intensification after fat grafting remains another restriction.

Instead, we all agree that harvested adipose tissue is composed of oil, mature adipocytes, extracellular matrix, watery components, and most important and critical for the survival of the graft, the SVF.

Indeed, when enriched with ATSCs (included in the SVF), lipotransfer has been associated with better graft viability and surgical cosmetic outcome for a longer time.

Regarding the evaluative conclusion between superficial adipose tissue (SAT) and deep adipose tissue (DAT) collected from human donors undergoing

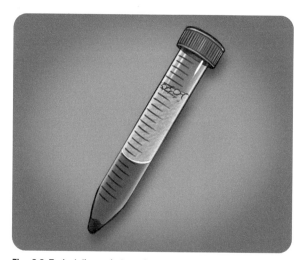

Fig. 9.6 Typical lipoaspirates after light centrifugation. Before the modern stromal vascular fraction procedure, maximum care was taken to collect the "white ring": the fat stroma (collagen) and the very bottom collection of the blood solid parts of the centrifuged fat.

the first-time liposuction for penis enlargement purposes, results revealed that SAT was homogeneously present in all body areas, whereas DAT was more abundant in the abdomen, hip, knee, peritrochanteric area, upper inner thigh, and posterior compartment of the arm. The SVF cell fraction from abdominal SAT lipoaspirates showed higher viability and the denser display of both stem/stromal surface antigen, endoglin (CD105) and the very important vascular endothelial growth factor (VEGF) when compared with DAT from the same harvesting site. Largely, SAT was associated with better stem properties, thus suggesting its preferable use as a donor site.

Still, strong controversy exists regarding the size of the cannula, the number of the import holes, the application of negative pressure, and manual or mechanical harvesting.

Multiperforated cannulas help reduce pressure on each hole, decreasing damage to the fat cells during sample collection. Trivisonno et al. compared 2-mm- and 3-mm-diameter cannulas, both with 170 mm length and a rounded tip. The 2-mm cannula had five round spirally placed ports, each with a 1-mm diameter, and the 3-mm cannula had a single side-located 3×9 mm port. The 2-mm cannula concurrently facilitated harvesting from more superficial and vascularized layers of adipose tissue, and reduced patient discomfort and trauma. In addition, the collected lipoaspirates from this 2-mm cannula were able to isolate more ATSCs, with a higher potential for capillary-like structure formation than the 3-mm cannula. Nevertheless, this was comparable only to the number of isolated ATSCs. All the other factors such as viability, morphology, and proliferation capacity of the fat did not vary significantly between the two cannulas.

Donor-site morbidity, such as a hematoma or, more frequently, local deformities caused by liposuction for penis enlargement and recipient-site complications, such as infections and, although extremely unlikely, pulmonary embolism, cardiac arrest, or deep venous thrombosis, represent zero disadvantages of adipose tissue transplant to the penis. Thus autologous fat grafting is reported to be a very safe procedure with very low morbidity. Malformation in the penis is rare, although official statistical data are missing, as such impediments are not reported, mainly because of

fear or shame; the most experienced and ethical well-trained doctor is a guarantee for fewer malformations and complications.

Results are enhanced when after 6 months, a second procedure is done. In the penis, anatomically, there is no fat present, but with the second procedure there is already a thin layer of fat in the grafted area, not only making it easier to inject, but also improving fat retention in the area.

Lipoaspirate centrifugation (3 minutes at 200 rev/min) is followed by a fat preparation process that produces a fat mix. During this process, fat is passed through one syringe into another, many times, in a gentle manner, through a syringe connector. This fat preparation process is done to (a) divide bigger particles of the lipoaspirate into smaller ones, (b) break the stromal connective tissue present between the fat cells, (c) mechanically make the fat particles as small as possible for smoother injection, preventing lake deposits and leaving a uniform final appearance, (d) make a smooth mix of the meshed collagen fibrils and the lipoaspirate (meshed collagen is added immediately after the fat centrifugation process to the mix). With this fat preparation process, we are deploying, dividing, and breaking the fat cell particles into smaller ones, obtaining a larger total surface area of fat cells.

I use accredited (FDA, ISO, CE, APPROVED) bovine collagen fibrils that are used in other non plastic surgery procedures where there is a need for enrichment of the receiving area for better formation on new connective collagen tissue and platelet adherence. You can find these with different trade names, you will see some of these brand names in the result section. In our practice, since 2006, for penis enlargement we most often use Lyostypt® (B Braun, Melsungen, Germany), which is only made of collagen fibrils of bovine origin (FDA, ISO, CE, and others approved), The fleece structure, being rich in collagen on the surface, offers an ideal framework for the adherence of platelets and for most of the PRP or PPP elements. We mix the finely meshed bovine collagen fibrils with the lipoaspirate small fat particles processed in-house. We inject this into the penis through the lipocannula. which has already been used to inject the PRP with the remaining PPP plus SVF.

All the structural elements adhere to the fat and the collagen fibrous network, offering the best layer for new fat cell growth, eventually with the main support of the SVF.

Tunneling

Maybe the most significant and principal important step for the outcome of the whole operation is the tunneling of the whole shaft of the penis. Using the same cannula as for the lipoaspiration, we perform a wide and complete undermining of the penile skin from the underlining tissue. This is the most important step of the whole procedure; if it is not done in the proper way by means of complete subcutaneous tunneling to the entire penis shaft, practically a controlled degloving, this could be the weak point for the outcome. We must take special consideration to not traumatize the far end where the foreskin (prepuce) is, but at the same time create an equal bed to accommodate the fat graft. Of extreme help to the correct tunneling is the previously injected PRP SVF.

Proper tunneling can be done by using the same cannula that was used for harvesting.

As soon as possible after the tunneling and the PRP, SVF, PPP liquid solution injection, the already final processed fat will be placed with the same syringe used to harvest, and will be injected through the same tunneling incision into the tunnel-network to the whole undermined area from the base to the prepuce of the

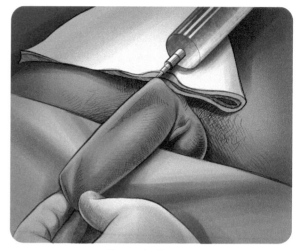

Fig. 9.8 Fat injection.

penis by means of light pressure in the syringe and diffuse instillation.

This whole procedure happens in a very short time, minutes if possible, as all the elements to be injected have already been prepared during the in-house procedure.

Attention should be paid after the injection to distributing the injected fat equally by means of long but gentle massaging. The fat goes into the tunnels and allocates similarly under the whole undermined area. Special care should be taken to distribute it uniformly, with no lumps or blank areas, up to the prepuce.

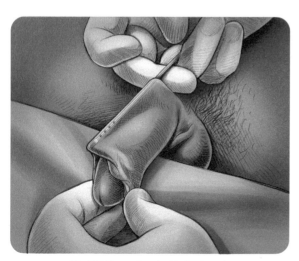

Fig. 9.7 Thorough and widening tunnel.

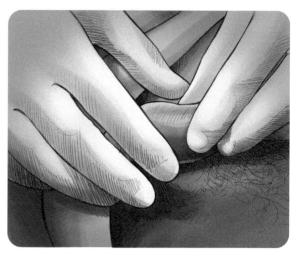

Fig. 9.9 Massaging to smooth the fat after injection.

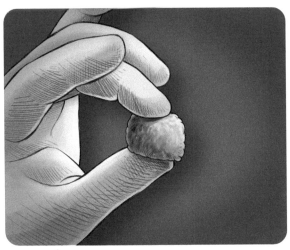

Fig. 9.10 If we mix fat with platelet-rich plasma in vitro, in 10 minutes, we will have a sponge-like solid product consisting of fat cells and fibrin.

The patient should be strongly advised to follow this same manipulation several times per day for the next 2–3 days.

It is not advisable to mix the fat before injection, with the PRP, SVF factors, or with any other endogenous factors. If you do that, within a few minutes (depending on the temperature), the fat organizes into a spongelike structure, becoming useless for injection.

TABLE 9.1	
Perforation of the prepuce, during operation	6
Subcutaneous infection of the shaft after the 10th postop day	1
Penile edema of more than 3 weeks	10
Fat nodules, fat lumps	12
Dehiscence	1
Delayed wound healing in the pubis wound area	10
Scarring	7
Penile deformity, sclerosing lipogranuloma, curvature	8
No increase in girth at all, fat necrosis	8
Keloids, scrotalization, disfiguring advancement of suprapubic hairy skin, different erection angle	None

We can use only PPP to dilute SVF and the mixture can be injected freely at the end, before the massaging. Remember that the PRP has been injected at the very beginning to work as a separator of the outer layers and nutrient to the injected fat.

We rarely perform the classical V–Y skin resection and the suspensory ligament detachment at the same time, as we believe that this type of operation does not offering anything to the enlargement, and adverse events and complications can happen.

CAN YOU SHARE WITH US ANY COMPLICATIONS?

Adverse events: All the side effects or complications were minor. None threatened the anatomical and functional integrity of the penis or the overall life/health of any of those individuals in whom the procedure was performed. Our complication rate was 7.5%.

CAN YOU SUMMARIZE YOUR FOLLOW-UP?

A total of 1399 fat transfers were performed; 850 during the period 1989–2006 and 549 during the period 2007–2019.

From 1989 to 2019, we have treated a total of 750 individuals using the same technique and protocol, divided into two chronological groups from 1989 to 2005 with 310 cases and from 2006 to 2019 with 440 cases. All were performed in our hospital or in a satellite clinic functioning as a day-surgery facility. The reason of this chronological division before and after 2006 is the fact that after that year, we used the meshed bovine fibrils and SVF.

Of 101 individuals who had only one attempt, 51 declared they were pleased with the results; 20 did not express any satisfaction or complaint, but felt that it was not worthwhile (either economically or because of the result itself) to undergo a second attempt and the other 30 individuals were lost to follow-up.

A total of 360 underwent a second operation after an average of 7 months (3 months to 2.5 years). Of these, 260 said they were satisfied to extremely satisfied, whereas 40 felt that the second operation did not meet their expectations and 60 were lost to follow-up.

A total of 210 individuals had a third attempt and 180 of them declared it was worth doing this third operation; 25 did not return again; and 5 claimed the third operation was not worth it.

Forty-five individuals underwent a fourth operation, of which 32 declared themselves to be happy with this fourth attempt, and 13 were lost to follow-up.

Thirty-four individuals had a fifth attempt, of which 18 were happy, 12 asked for a sixth operation, and 4 did not return.

Also, during the first period, the overall satisfaction was less, as we had to do a greater number of repeat procedures. During the second period, when we gradually started applying PRP, SVF, ATSCs, together with the bovine collagen fibrils, the rate of repetitions was lowered and the satisfaction rate increased.

WHY DO YOU THINK THIS TECHNIQUE SHOULD BE IN THE ARMAMENTARIUM OF ANY PLASTIC SURGEON?

Any plastic surgeon should have a thorough knowledge of and be familiar with this technique. It should be offered in their practice, as penis enlargement is becoming more popular every day, and thousands of male individuals are seeking help to satisfy their desire. If we as plastic surgeons do not do it, and do it well, patients can end up in the hands of unscrupulous providers who will not advise the right treatments, with disastrous, undesirable results that can even cause permanent damage to the male genital structure.

WHAT TIPS CAN YOU GIVE US TO INCLUDE THIS PROCEDURE IN OUR PRACTICE?

The best technique is the one that each of us knows best and feels more secure in proceeding with.

Complete and efficient tunneling perhaps is the key to the success of the penis enlargement procedure.

Expert Profile

Theodore Vodoukis
Plastic Surgeon
Athens, Greece

EDUCATION

- Languages: Fluent in English, Greek, and Italian.
- Graduated in 1975 from the Athens University Medical School.
- Board Certified General Surgeon, 1979.
- Board Certified Plastic Surgeon, 1982.
- ECFMG diploma since 1980.

- FACS (Fellow, American College of Surgeons) since 1987.
- GMC (General Medical Council) member, UK, since 1980.
- GMC registered Principal Specialty List, Surgeon and Plastic Surgeon.

ACADEMIC

- Internship, Athens University Department of General Surgery, 1979.
- PhD, Cum Laude from Athens University Medical School, Microsurgery—Hemodynamics, 1981.
- Visiting professor at NYU Sachs Institute, 1985–1988.
- Professor of Aesthetic Plastic Surgery at Western Athens University, 1990–2012.
- Chair, National Secretaries of ISAPS (International Society of Aesthetic Plastic Surgery), 2006–2012.
- Founding member of the ISPRES (International Society of Plastic Regenerative Surgery).
- Member of the Educational Academy of the IPRAS (International Confederation of Plastic Reconstructive Aesthetic Surgery).
- Participation in more than 115 international conventions, of which more than 25 were as chair on round tables, 44 publications, scientific magazines, and educational publications.
- Member, International Medical Committee, FIA (Federation International de Automobile).

WORK EXPERIENCE

1975–1979: Internship at the Athens National University Surgical Clinic.

1979–1981: Captain (OF-2), in the Hellenic Army Medical Corps.

1981–1985: Registrar and Senior Registrar at the St. Lawrence Chepstow and St. Thomas' Hospital, London.

1985–1988: Private practice, fellow with Yves Gerard Ylouz, Athens – Paris – Bologna.

1988–2014: Chair and head of the Plastic Surgery Unit at MITERA Hospital, Athens, Greece.

2014–Present: Consultant at Rea Maternity Hospital, IASO Hospital.

1984–Present: Owner of private practice and consulting firm, "MEDICART"

1975–Present: FIA Chief Medical Officer (WRC, ERC, F1 races) – member of the Medical Committee and Anti-Doping Disciplinary Committee.

SPECIAL INTERESTS

- Radio operator's License – Amateur, SV1DJ.
- Automobile racing with international distinctions.

BIBLIOGRAPHY

Ansell Research. The penis size survey. March 2001. http://esvc000171.wic049u.server-web.com/education/research.htm 30.

Cancello R, Zulian A, Gentilini D, et al: Molecular and morphologic characterization of superficial- and deep-subcutaneous adipose tissue subdivisions in human obesity, *Obesity (Silver Spring)*. 21:2562–2570, 2013.

Center for Program Evaluation and Performance Management, Bureau of Justice Assistance. Biased sample, Glossary. Archived from the original on 8 September 2015. Available from: BJA.gov.

Chen J, Gefen A, Greenstein A, Matzkin H, Elad D: Predicting penile size during erection, *Int J Impot Res*. 12:328–333, 2001.

Coskun H, Summerfield TL, Kniss DA, Friedman A: Mathematical modeling of preadipocyte fate determination, *J Theor Biol*. 265:87–94, 2010.

Cypess AM, Lehman S, Williams G, et al: Identification and importance of brown adipose tissue in adult humans, *New Engl J Med*. 360:1509–1517, 2009.

Fried SK, Lee MJ, Karastergiou K: Shaping fat distribution: new insights into the molecular determinants of depot- and sex-dependent adipose biology, *Obesity (Silver Spring)*. 23(7):1345–1352, 2015.

Kelley DE, Thaete FL, Troost F, Huwe T, Goodpaster BH: Subdivisions of subcutaneous abdominal adipose tissue and insulin resistance, *Am J Physiol Endocrinol Metab*. 278:E941–E948, 2000.

Kim WW: History and cultural perspective. In Park NC, Moon DG, Kim SW, editors: *Penile Augmentation*, Berlin, Germany, 2016, Springer, pp 11–26.

Markman B, Barton FE Jr: Anatomy of the subcutaneous tissue of the trunk and lower extremity, *Plast Reconstr Surg*. 80:248–254, 1987.

Nguyen A, Guo J, Banyard DA, et al: Stromal vascular fraction: a regenerative reality? Part 1: current concepts and review of the literature, *J Plast Reconstr Aesthetic Surg*. 69:170–179, 2016.

Pagnotti GM, Styner M: Exercise regulation of marrow adipose tissue, *Front Endocrinol (Lausanne)*. 7:94, 2016.

Panfilov DE: Augmentative phalloplasty, *Aesthetic Plast Surg*. 30:183–197, 2006.

Park JK, Doo AR, Kim JH, et al: Prospective investigation of penile length with newborn male circumcision and second to fourth digit ratio, *Can Urol Assoc J*. 10:E296–E299, 2016.

Ponchietti R, Mondaini N, Bonafè M, Di Loro F, Biscioni S, Masieri L: Penile length and circumference: a study on 3,300 young Italian males, *Eur Urol* 39:183–186, 2001.

Promodu K, Shanmughadas KV, Bhat S, Nair KR: Penile length and circumference: an Indian study, *Int J Impot Res*. 19:558–563, 2007.

Ramakrishna S, Tian L, Wang C, et al: Quality management systems for medical device manufacture. In Ramakrishna S, Tian L, Wang C, et al, editors: *Medical Devices: Regulations, Standards and Practices. Woodhead Publishing Series in Biomaterials 103*, Elsevier, 2015, pp 49–64.

Robert P: *Fat, Fighting the Obesity Epidemic*, Oxford, 2015, Oxford University Press, 68.

Rosique RG, Rosique MJF, De Moraes CG: Gluteoplasty with autologous fat tissue, *Plast Reconstr Surg*. 135:1381–1389, 2015.

Smith P, Adams WP Jr, Lipschitz AH, et al: Autologous human fat grafting: effect of harvesting and preparation techniques on adipocyte graft survival, *Plast Reconstr Surg*. 117:1836–1844, 2006.

Stang J, Story M: Adolescent growth and development. In Stang J, Story M, editors: *Guidelines for Adolescent Nutrition Services*, University of Minnesota, 2005, pp 3.

Stoltz JF, de Isla N, Li YP, et al: Stem cells and regenerative medicine: myth or reality of the 21st century, *Stem Cells Int*. 2015:734731, 2015.

Tchoukalova YD, Votruba SB, Tchkonia T, Giorgadze N, Kirkland JL, Jensen MD: Regional differences in cellular mechanisms of adipose tissue gain with overfeeding, *Proc Natl Acad Sci U S A*. 107:18226–18231, 2010.

Veale D, Miles S, Bramley S, Muir G, Hodsoll J: Am 1 normal? A systematic review and construction of nomograms for flaccid and erect penis length and circumference in up to 15 521 men, *BJU Int*. 115:978–986, 2015.

Wessells H, Lue TF, McAninch JW: Penile length in the flaccid and erect states: guidelines for penile augmentation, *J Urol*. 156:995–997, 1996.

Wylie KR, Eardley I: Penile size and the 'small penis syndrome,' *BJU Int*. 99(6):1449–1455, 2007.

Zuk PA, Zhu M, Ashjian P, et al: Human adipose tissue is a source of multipotent stem cells, *Mol Biol Cell*. 13:4279–4295, 2002.

Facial Gender Differences in Nonsurgical Treatments and Treatment of the Tear Trough Deformity

Lina Triana Invited Expert Fabian Cortinas

Plastic Surgeon, Cali, Colombia, Buenos Aires, Argentina

Chapter Outline

Why Offer Nonsurgical Treatments? Male and Female Differences

Males

Females

Why Is it Important as Doctors to Have Different Treatment Approaches Between Male and Female Patients?

Important Anatomical Differences Between Males and Females

Differences in Nonsurgical Facial Assessment Between Males and Females

Overall appearance/skin

Head overview

Facial thirds

Soft tissues and bony structure

Treatment Plan: Pigmentation

Treatment Plan: Wrinkles

Botulinum Toxin: How to Avoid Feminizing a Male

Masseters and Botulinum Toxin

Treatment Plan: Fillers

Filler treatment plan for females

Filler treatment plan for males

Expert Approach: Treating the Tear Trough Deformity: Taking Away a Tired Look or Fat Bags Without Surgery

Why did you decide to do this technique?

When did you learn it or if it is your own, how did you end up doing it?

Can this technique be compared to others and why?

What do you consider to be important landmarks and anatomy to be able to better perform this technique?

Can you explain to us how you do the assessment on a patient asking for this procedure?

Can you give us some guidelines for constructing an assessment chart?

Can you describe your technique?

How can we avoid complications?

Can you summarize your follow-up and patient recommendations?

Why do you think this technique should be in the armamentarium of any plastic surgeon?

What tips can you give us to include this procedure in our practice and How to market it?

Expert Profile

What did Steve Jobs do for Apple? He did something different. He brought to a technology company the concept that design, and how a product is presented, are important. Before him, any computer you bought was just the same boring design; what the technology companies centered on was what was inside that computer, but Steve Jobs proved with Apple that design and presentation make a difference.

So, what connection does he have with facial aesthetics? We must never forget our face is our presentation card, the first impression others have of us. How we look helps us in our interaction with others and in our relationships. This is why aesthetic procedures are more and more popular in today's world. And this is why the concept that beauty helps us escalate in our life, and in our career, proves true every day.

Looking good does count, as *Forbes* magazine proved CEOs earn more money when they are better looking. Studies at the University of Texas also showed that an attractive person can earn 3%–4% more than a less attractive peer. In another study, the University of Chicago showed that the more attractive a person is, the more confidence they have in themselves, and the better performance they show in all aspects of their lives.

Also, good design is shown as being glamorous and makes any product look more important and desirable, becoming itself an aspirational buy. This is what we as human beings, in this world, consciously or unconsciously, are seeking. Coming back to us humans, what makes us wanted by others? What make us look like an aspirational catch? Here I am not just referring to how the opposite sex or a future partner sees us, but how corporations see us, how even our own patients see us. The better design we have, the more aspirational we will be for others. Here it is obvious that males and females have clear differences in their structure; we carry preconceptions of male and female appearances, and how we (as men or women) want others to see us. Today, males and females do not necessarily have different goals, but it is clear in the end our sex does not matter, as each individual has his/her specific goal, one he/she owns. This is why I always like to come back to the essence. It is crucial to have the knowledge of the structural differences between a man and a woman, but we must listen to our patients to be able to construct the best treatment for him/her at a specific time and place.

We as surgeons often might want to do a great surgical technique that is just right for this patient, but it is up to the patient to decide if they want to have it or not. Today, it is not like before, where patients came to our office saying, "Doctor, what you think is best for me? You are the specialist." More and more today, patients are participating actively in their treatment decisions. Because of easy access to information and techniques of today, patients just think they are surgeons already and many come not just asking, but with a demanding attitude: "This is what I want you to do on me," and if they are not pleased, they will simply go to another doctor. Here, my friends, is where we as doctors need to remember our Hippocratic Oath,

which says always give the best to our patients and never harm them.

So, how do you succeed in creating the best possible treatment plan for the patient? Well, if the patient is seeking a nonsurgical option and he/she needs a surgical approach according, to your assessment, then be clear about realistic expectations of the nonsurgical option, but never insist if they state from the beginning they do not want surgery.

Today, we are always running out of time. To have some days off has become a luxury for many, so when you have some free time, you need to weigh up to see how time can be better spent, in leisure time, with family, or in recovery from a surgical procedure.

It is also well known that in aesthetic procedures, we do not make molds and in particular, we can never attempt to use the same approach and treatment plan for males and females. Here are some important observations to bear in mind during a consultation.

Why Offer Nonsurgical Treatments? Male and Female Differences

MALES

- Are more likely to not seek a huge change.
- Do not like others to know they had an aesthetic procedure.
- Prefer no downtime.
- Are more impatient.
- Have a better income to continue coming regularly for nonsurgical options.
- See surgery as something more extreme.
- Are more afraid of surgery.

FEMALES

- Are more prone to share with their girlfriends that they had a procedure done.
- Socialize more their concerns with others before making the decision to visit a specialist.
- Tend to come with a specific idea of what they want.
- Tend to have a fixed result in their minds; may even bring a picture of how they want to look after the procedure, "just like her."
- Are more spontaneous, impulsive buyers, so can end up having a procedure that is not best for them or that is not in the best place to be done.

They can end up having the procedure done by a nonspecialist doctor.
- Have more patience with the recovery period.
- Are more willing to have some downtime.

Why Is it Important as Doctors to Have Different Treatment Approaches Between Male and Female Patients?

Because males want to be more private than women, a more private setting must be constructed when wanting to captivate male clients.

Women are more prone to wait for longer periods; they will wait longer for you in the waiting room. However, you need to be really sharp on the agenda with men, as they are not willing to wait for you, even if you are the best doctor.

You need to be more data-oriented with males, share more scientific data with them, less of a selling approach. Females want more what is a trending today and what their friends have had done.

Females want to be prettier, more seductive and younger, to not show their age. Males want to be more masculine and better than their contenders; also they want to look younger.

Important Anatomical Differences Between Males and Females

There are important anatomical differences between males and females. Dividing them in areas will facilitate the delivery of information to you. We will start giving a general view where we can see how the skull is bulkier in males and rounder in females. Now we will divided into 3 areas:

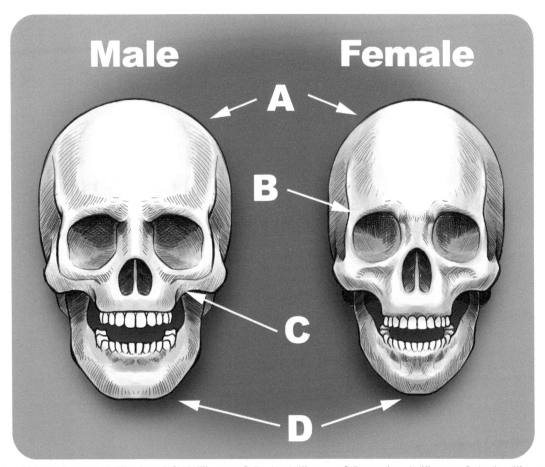

Fig. 10.1 Male and female skull differences. A: Skull differences. B: Forehead differences. C: Zygomatic arch differences. D: Jawline differences.

TABLE 10.1	Important Anatomical Differences Between Males and Females
Skull	The male skull is heavier and bulkier; the female skull is rounder and less prominent.
Forehead	Males have a rounder forehead and females a flatter one. Regarding the supraorbital rim, there is a great distinction between males and females, which is that males have a rounder and more prominent supraorbital region and superciliary arch than females.
Zygomatic arch	This is more prominent in males than in females.
Jawline	Males have a more defined and wider jawline and mandibular angle, with more prominent masseter muscles than females.

the forehead, the zygomatic and the jawline. The forehead area is normally rounder in males and flatter in females, and where going down towards the supraorbital rim, the supraciliary arch in males is much more prominent than in females. In contrast the zygomatic region is more prominent in females than in males. And the jawline in males is wider, with a more prominent masseter muscle and more definition at the mandibular angle than in females.

Differences in Nonsurgical Facial Assessment Between Males and Females

OVERALL APPEARANCE/SKIN

It is important to have a regular skin tone for a better overall appearance and optimal result with our non-surgical treatment approach.

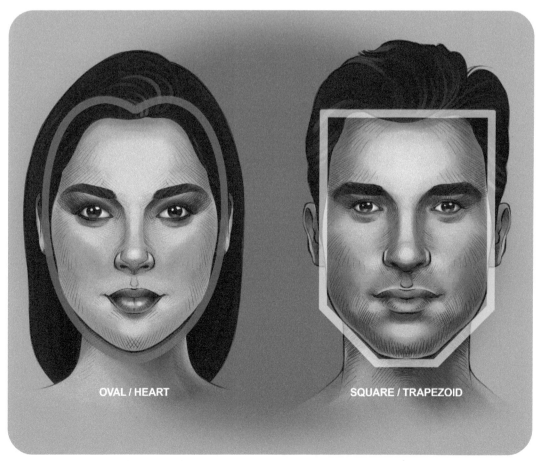

Fig. 10.2 Facial shape differences in males and females. Females are more oval and heart shaped and males are more square and trapezoid.

Females tend to have more hyperpigmented skin secondary to hormonal changes and dark spots distributed irregularly through their face than men. If this is the case, it is important to include a depigmentation option in the treatment plan.

Males tend to have more open pores and their skin tends to be oilier, so cleaning routines must be included in their treatment plan.

Females' skin tend to be thinner and more prone to dehydration, so good hydration and skin thickening options must be included in their treatment plan.

Females tend to be more aware of their wrinkles, so options to prevent or minimize them must be included in their treatment plan.

HEAD OVERVIEW

Face shape in males tends to be more squarish or trapezoid and in females, more oval or heart shaped; the younger the woman is, the more inverted triangle shape she has.

When a female face that is too square or a male face that is not trapezoid is found during the consultation, treatment options to counteract these facial shapes must be included.

Hair is very important for males and females. In females, hair loss tends to be more generalized all over their scalp but in men, it is more evident, especially as the hairline starts to recede, particularly at the temples, and hair loss is greater in certain areas such as the corona. When hair loss is identified during the assessment, it is a must to include hair-loss treatment options.

FACIAL THIRDS
SOFT TISSUES AND BONY STRUCTURE

Face shape in males tends to have more angles and in females, it is rounder, smoother, and curvier.

When a female face that lacks smoothness or a male face that is too curvy is found during the consultation, treatment options to counteract these facial shapes must be included.

Lips: We must lose our prejudice that prominent lips are only for women. For a male to be more masculine, it is essential to have a prominent lower third and the lips are crucial here. Many times, male lips share a protagonist role in males along with their squared mandible, especially their lower lip. If you are still not convinced, just have a look at famous good-looking

TABLE 10.2	Facial Thirds, Soft Tissues, and Bony Structure
Upper third	Forehead is wider in males than in females. Eyebrows are lower and straighter in males and higher and more arched in females.
Middle third	More prominent in females than in males.
Lower third	More square in males and rounder in females. Must be prominent in males.

men. They all have prominent lips in their prominent square faces.

Treatment Plan: Pigmentation

Mostly used in females, as they have more pigmentation problems. Females are more likely to accept no sun exposure and use of regular sunblock after treatment.

Depigmentation treatment options:
- Laser resurfacing
- Dermabrasion
- Chemical peel
- Creams

Treatment Plan: Wrinkles

More requested in females, but important to be included in male treatment plans.

Treatment options:
- Hydration creams
- Platelet-rich plasma
- Nonsurgical devices (lasers, radiofrequency, etc.)
- Low-density hyaluronic acids (HAs)
- Botulinum toxin

Botulinum Toxin: How to Avoid Feminizing a Male

Focus on preventing changes that can make eyebrows feminine.
- Prevent lateral eyebrow elevation. Do not add lower lateral eyelid injection.
- Examine the frontal muscle properly.

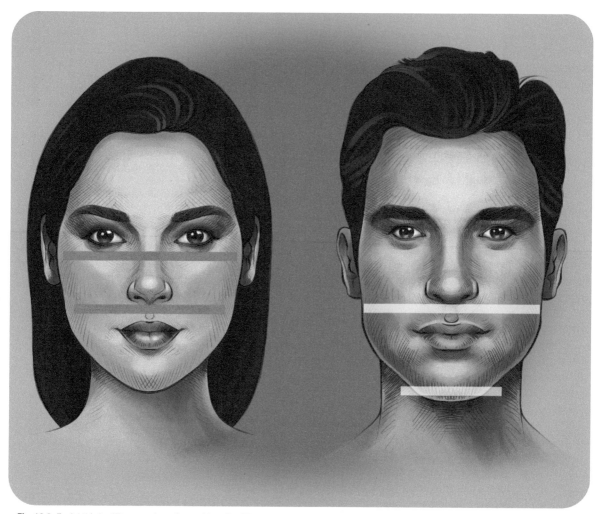

Fig. 10.3 Facial thirds differences in males and females. The more prominent area is the lower third in males and the middle third in females.

- Are wrinkles present lateral to the frontal crest? If yes, always add lateral to crest injections.
- These will prevent lateral elevation of the eyebrow.
- Prevent taking away too much force from corrugators and procerus.
  - This can separate interciliary distance, which can be tolerated in a female face but not in a male one.
  - Males tend to have fuller and more midline eyebrow connection.

When a wide forehead is present with receding hair in the temples, examine how high in the forehead the wrinkles go. If wrinkles are present in the temple area, make sure to add an injection point up there. If you do not do so, the patient will return saying, "Doctor, it looks like I have a pair of horns every time I move my forehead."

Masseters and Botulinum Toxin

A good option for demasculinizing a female face is to look for prominent masseter muscles and if present, add botulinum toxin to them, which will give a woman a rounder, less square lower third.

Be careful when a male comes asking for some botulinum toxin on their masseters to decrease bruxism. This can certainly help them with their condition, but can lessen a squarer and wider mandible angle, taking away masculine attributes.

Treatment Plan: Fillers

The most important factor on what filler to choose is that your body will be able to reabsorb it. Any substance that our bodies are not able to reabsorb is called a biopolymer and we must never inject biopolymers into our patients.

FILLER TREATMENT PLAN FOR FEMALES

As we live on planet Earth and planet Earth has a gravitational force, everything comes down with time. This is why the female face changes from being an inverted triangular shape when young to becoming a regular triangle with decreasing emphasis on the protagonist middle third found in females.

With this in mind, all efforts must be focused to add volume on the middle third in an attempt to elevate tissues that have fallen and prevent a lower third that is bulky and less female, less attractive.

This is why adding volume to the temples is also very useful for the female rejuvenation approach with fillers.

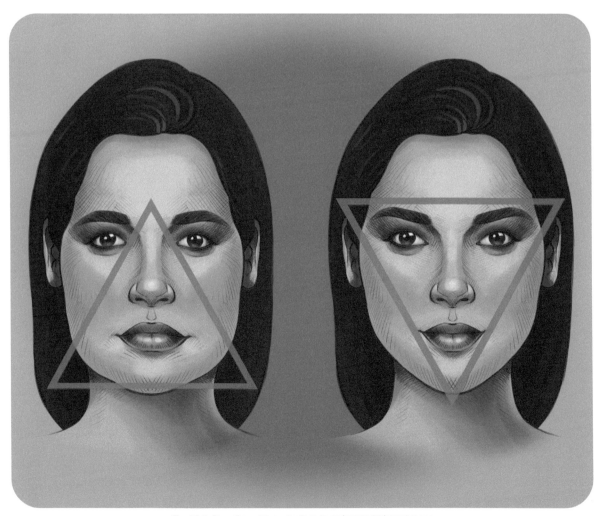

Fig. 10.4 Changing a triangular face to an inverted triangular one.

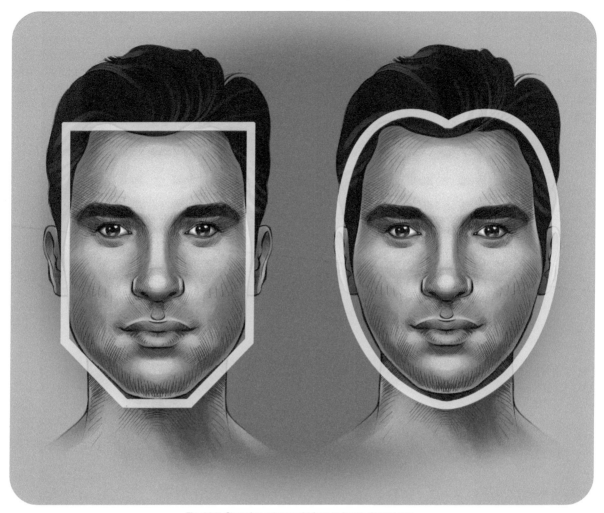

Fig. 10.5 Changing a trapezoid face to heart-shaped one.

Also, always add some volume on the middle chin to help build up a more inverted triangular V shape.

FILLER TREATMENT PLAN FOR MALES

As we usually add volume on the middle third of female faces to take away sagginess that shows on the lower third, this is what we tend to do in male faces too. This is why we must be very careful when injecting a man to prevent ending up with a prominent middle third and giving a too-rounded appearance. Remember, males do not have curves in their faces.

This is why in males, you should always add volume on the mandible angles and jawline and when wanting to lift the lower third, stay away from the middle third center. When injecting a male middle third, always make sure to equilibrate it with the width of the mandibular angle. Remember, we need to end up with a square face.

Expert Approach: Treating the Tear Trough Deformity: Taking Away a Tired Look or Fat Bags Without Surgery

Fabian Cortiñas
Plastic Surgeon
Buenos Aires, Argentina

Dr. Fabian Cortiñas is an internationally renowned surgeon who shares all over the world his expertise in the field of nonsurgical injectable treatments to enhance and rejuvenate the face. Here, he gives us tips on how to take away the tired look of fat bags with a nonsurgical approach.

WHY DID YOU DECIDE TO DO THIS TECHNIQUE?

When I started with fillers using several different types of products, HA was introduced to the market. Only one NASHA brand was available and showed good tolerance and adaptability to different regions. Its hydroscopic properties showed not only projection and voluminization (a new term coined at that time to explain the replacement of volume loss), but also it improved the quality of the overlying skin.

In order to treat small irregularities in the lower eyelid region and the orbital sulcus without adding volume to the cheeks, I started to fill small irregularities with diluted HA; 50% HA and 50% lidocaine 2% with epinephrine solution was used since 2007.

WHEN DID YOU LEARN IT OR IF IT IS YOUR OWN, HOW DID YOU END UP DOING IT?

I learned from personal experience regarding the use of fillers and HA products. After some time in a surgery-mainly practice, I saw a presentation from Steve Faigien, someone I have as a reference in periorbital treatments and from whom I learned many techniques, and this gave me courage to continue with it.

CAN THIS TECHNIQUE BE COMPARED TO OTHERS AND WHY?

Most procedures to add volume to the lower eyelid include the cheek area, and when the orbicular sulcus is treated, most of the proposals recommend deep injections under the orbicularis, applying regular products. What I usually do is a more superficial injection in the thickness of the muscle with the diluted HA in small aliquots two or three times for a complete correction.

WHAT DO YOU CONSIDER TO BE IMPORTANT LANDMARKS AND ANATOMY TO BE ABLE TO BETTER PERFORM THIS TECHNIQUE?

Surface anatomy. I am going to fill a defect that is visible and when the defect disappears, treatment is completed. We are not adding volume to the cheeks or to the lower eyelid; we just create an even surface between the lower eyelid and the cheek.

Quality of tissues is crucial because it is easy to create a bag with small amounts of product.

CAN YOU EXPLAIN TO US HOW YOU DO THE ASSESSMENT ON A PATIENT ASKING FOR THIS PROCEDURE?

Nowadays, I receive patients asking for this specific procedure because of word of mouth, but regular patients come to the office asking to get rid of their tired look, or dark circles, as they call it.

CAN YOU GIVE US SOME GUIDELINES FOR CONSTRUCTING AN ASSESSMENT CHART?

The ideal candidate is a young patient with an uneven surface between the lower eyelid and the cheek but when assessing the quality of the skin, we may include patients from different ages with good skin tone. However, we may offer a reasonable improvement to patients with bags who cannot afford surgery for many reasons.

CAN YOU DESCRIBE YOUR TECHNIQUE?

When assessing the patient with lighting from above and below in a sitting position, areas of shadow will show, making it easier to recognize irregularities such as the orbicularis sulcus shape and tear trough.

Dilute HA 50/50 is prepared with a connector. The skin is cleaned, and the injection is done very slowly, small aliquots into the deep sulcus, mid distance between the skin and periosteum. Undercorrection is preferable, three to four points of injections on each side and wait for 10 days. Most of the time, three sessions are enough, with 0.2–0.3 cc solution on each side. The final amount of HA used is usually very small and the correction may last many years.

HOW CAN WE AVOID COMPLICATIONS?

The procedure must be done with patience in a relaxed environment and the injection in a very slow motion, small amounts, while checking pain as a sign of vascular or nerve injury. Thirty percent of patients get some bruising that may last up to 1 week. The following session must be done without any residual bruising or inflammatory reaction.

CAN YOU SUMMARIZE YOUR FOLLOW-UP AND PATIENT RECOMMENDATIONS?

I check patients every 2 weeks until I find a complete correction. No special care is needed after each session.

WHY DO YOU THINK THIS TECHNIQUE SHOULD BE IN THE ARMAMENTARIUM OF ANY PLASTIC SURGEON?

Because plastic surgeons are the most prepared to lead nonsurgical procedures, fillers add patients to the consultation, and finally because is a tool to correct small defects, even ones that may be present after surgery.

WHAT TIPS CAN YOU GIVE US TO INCLUDE THIS PROCEDURE IN OUR PRACTICE AND HOW TO MARKET IT?

The best way to market it is to educate patients that there is a nonsurgical option for correction of eyelid bags and also in young people to take away a tired look.

Expert Profile

Fabian Cortiñas
Plastic Surgeon
Buenos Aires, Argentina

Dr. Cortiñas went to Medical School in Rosario, his home town, and after finishing his training in general surgery, he moved to Buenos Aires to undertake a postgraduate course in plastic surgery at El Salvador University.

From 1996 to date, he works in his own office in Buenos Aires with emphasis on aesthetic surgical and nonsurgical treatments.

He is a member of SALTEM, an Argentine Society for Lasers and Medical Technologies, and is medical director of IMQ BA, an institute with one of the most important laser centers in South America.

Dr. Cortiñas is active member of the Argentine Society of Plastic Surgery (SACPER), the Buenos Aires Plastic Surgery Society (SCPBA), the American Society for Aesthetic Plastic Surgery (ASAPS), and the International Society of Aesthetic Plastic Surgery (ISAPS). He has been a board member and committee member of SACPER, SCPBA, SALTEM, and ISAPS.

His academic background includes lectures at many plastic surgery congresses. Some of the latest conferences have been in France, Spain, USA, South Korea, Vietnam, Japan, and Brazil. He is the author of publications in the *ASJ* and a book chapter, which is in process.

His philosophy and approach to facial aesthetics is about proportions and harmony, with a deep respect for the patient's natural anatomy. Facial implants are a great tool in the armamentarium to improve proportions, but are frequently applied in large amounts with a consequent increased risk of side effects and complications. Efforts must be made to obtain the best result with the smallest amount of filler possible.

BIBLIOGRAPHY

Fitzgerald R, Graivier MH, Kane M, et al: Facial aesthetic analysis, *Aesthet Surg J.* 30(Suppl):25S–27S, 2010.

Gibelli D, Codari M, Rosati R, et al: A quantitative analysis of lip aesthetics: the influence of gender and aging, *Aesthetic Plast Surg.* 39(5):771–776, 2015.

Harrar H, Myers S, Ghanem AM: Art or science? An evidence-based approach to human facial beauty: a quantitative analysis towards an informed clinical aesthetic practice, *Aesthetic Plast Surg.* 42:137–146, 2018.

Linkiv G, Mally P, Czyz CN, et al: Quantification of the aesthetic desirable female midface position, *Aesthet Surg J.* 38(3):231–240, 2017.

Viana GAP, Osaki MH, Cariello AJ, et al: Treatment of tear trough deformity with hyaluronic acid, *Aesthet Surg J.* 31(2):225–231, 2011.

Index

Page numbers followed by "*f*" indicate figures

A

Abdominoplasty
  extended, 7*f*, 8*f*
  ultrasonic liposuction-assisted high lateral
      tension, 2

B

Body contouring
  anatomical differences, males *vs.* females, 2
  CAP abdominoplasty, 6*f*
  complications, 3, 10
  definition, 2
  epigastric laxity, 5*f*
  extended abdominoplasty, 7*f*, 8*f*
  follow-up and patient recommendations, 11
  guidelines, assessment chart, 7
  Klein solution, 9*f*
  landmarks and anatomy, 3
  preoperative and postoperative anterior view, 4*f*
  rectus fascia plication, 10*f*
  superficial and deep fascias, 9
  treatment approaches, 2
  ultrasonic liposuction assisted high lateral tension
      abdominoplasty technique, 2
  wound healing, 11
Brambilla, Massimiliano, 38
Breast implants
  approaches, 20
  importance, 20
  mastopexy technique, 20
    approximation and suturing, 22, 23*f*
    basal compensating triangles, 21*f*
    complications, 28
    dog ears correction, 26*f*
    en-bloc explantation, 25
    follow-up and patient recommendations, 28
    free-hand technique, 23
    implant removal and, 24, 25*f*
    landmarks and anatomy, 23
    vs. original technique, 23
    periareolar incision, 20, 21*f*
    pinching maneuver, 21*f*
    preoperative markings, 29*f*, 29, 30*f*, 31*f*
    risk of spontaneous rupture, 28
    secondary repositioning, 27
    vascular areolar impairment, 27*f*
    vertical limits, skin resection, 21*f*

C

Caminer, David, 61, 64, 71
Campiglio, Gianluca, 30
Citarella, Enzo, 57, 60
Clitoris hood insertion, 40, 42*f*. *See also*
      Hoodplasty
Cortiñas, Fabian, 100

D

Dartos fascia, 57
Depigmentation, 94

E

Episiotomy scar treatment, 34, 35*f*

F

Fat grafting, 76
Females, facial gender differences
  anatomical differences, 93
  facial shape differences, 95*f*
  facial thirds differences, 96*f*
  fillers, 97*f*, 97
  head overview, 93
  nonsurgical treatments, 92
  overall appearance/skin, 93
  patient recommendations, 100
  pigmentation, 94
  skull differences, 94*f*
  soft tissues and bony structure, 93
  treatment approaches, 93
  wrinkles, 95

G

G-spot enhancer procedures, 41
Gynoplasty surgery, 34

H

Hoodplasty
  assessment, 42
  complications, 44
  follow-up, 44

Hoodplasty (*Cont.*)
  horseshoe resection, 43, 44*f*
  vs. labia minora resection, 42
  vs. labiaplasty, 40
  landmarks and anatomy, 42
  longitudinal resection, 43
  non-surgical aesthetic genital procedures, 41
  plication of clitoris body, 43
  procedure, 44
  reasons for, 39
Horseshoe resection, hoodplasty, 43, 44*f*
Hymenoplasty, 41

I
Inevitable scar
  vaginal surgery, 33
  vulvar surgery, 33

J
J-plasma technology, liposuction, 13, 16
  complications, 16
  importance, 14
  landmarks and anatomy, 15
  patient assessment, 15
  procedure, 15
  recommendations, 16
  vs. VASER, 15

L
Labia majora plasty, 40
Labia minora size reduction, 41
Labiaplasty, 40
Liposculpture, 13
Liposuction
  J-plasma technology, 13, 16
    complications, 16
    importance, 14
    landmarks and anatomy, 15
    patient assessment, 15
    procedure, 15
    recommendations, 16
    vs. VASER, 15
  power-assisted machine, 13
  Renuvion, 13
  superficial, 13
  VASER, 13

M
Males, facial gender differences
  anatomical differences, 93
  assessment chart, 99

  botulinum toxin, 96
    masseters and, 97
  complications, 99
  facial shape differences, 95*f*
  facial thirds differences, 96*f*
  fillers, 98*f*, 98
  head overview, 93
  nonsurgical treatments, 92
  overall appearance/skin, 93
  patient recommendations, 100
  pigmentation, 94
  skull differences, 94*f*
  soft tissues and bony structure, 93
  treatment approaches, 93
  wrinkles, 95
Mastopexy technique, breast implants, 20
  approximation and suturing, 22, 23*f*
  basal compensating triangles, 21*f*
  complications, 28
  dog ears correction, 26*f*
  en-bloc explantation, 25
  follow-up and patient recommendations, 28
  free-hand technique, 23
  implant removal and, 24, 25*f*
  landmarks and anatomy, 23
  vs. original technique, 23
  periareolar incision, 20, 21*f*
  pinching maneuver, 21*f*
  preoperative markings, 29*f*, 29, 30*f*, 31*f*
  risk of spontaneous rupture, 28
  secondary repositioning, 27
  vascular areolar impairment, 27*f*
  vertical limits, skin resection, 21*f*
Miradmi, Wafaa, 17
Mons pubis, 40

P
Penile lengthening procedures, 63
  advantages of harvesting fat, 64
  assessment, 66
  complications, 64, 68
  dermal fat grafting, 65
  follow-up and patient recommendations, 68
  landmarks and anatomy, 65
  penile scrotal webbing, 70*f*, 70
  scrotal reduction, 69*f*, 69
  V-Y advancement flap, 64, 66*f*, 67
Penile scrotal webbing, 70*f*, 70
  markings, 70*f*
  postoperative, 70*f*
  resultant scar after, 70*f*